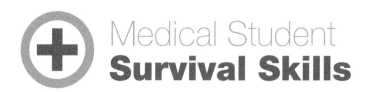

ECG

T0261900

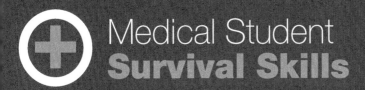

Medical Student
Survival Skills

ECG

Philip Jevon RN BSc(Hons) PGCE
Academy Manager/Tutor
Walsall Teaching Academy, Manor Hospital, Walsall, UK

Jayant Gupta FRCP
Consultant Cardiologist, Senior Academy Tutor
Walsall Healthcare NHS Trust, Manor Hospital, Walsall, UK

Consulting Editors

Jonathan Pepper BMedSci BM BS FRCOG MD
FAcadMEd
Consultant Obstetrics and Gynaecology, Head of Academy
Walsall Healthcare NHS Trust, Manor Hospital, Walsall, UK

Jamie Coleman MBChB MD MA(Med Ed)
FRCP FBPhS
Professor in Clinical Pharmacology and Medical Education / MBChB Deputy
  Programme Director
School of Medicine, University of Birmingham, Birmingham, UK

WILEY Blackwell

Registered Office(s)
John Wiley & Sons, Inc., 111 River Street, Hoboken, NJ 07030, USA
John Wiley & Sons Ltd, The Atrium, Southern Gate, Chichester, West Sussex, PO19 8SQ, UK

Editorial Office
9600 Garsington Road, Oxford, OX4 2DQ, UK

For details of our global editorial offices, customer services, and more information about Wiley products visit us at www.wiley.com.

Wiley also publishes its books in a variety of electronic formats and by print-on-demand. Some content that appears in standard print versions of this book may not be available in other formats.

Library of Congress Cataloging-in-Publication Data

Names: Jevon, Philip, author. | Gupta, Jayant, author.
Title: Medical student survival skills. ECG / Philip Jevon, Dr Jayant Gupta.
Other titles: ECG
Description: Hoboken, NJ : Wiley-Blackwell, 2020. | Includes bibliographical references and index. |
Identifiers: LCCN 2018060335 (print) | LCCN 2018061637 (ebook) | ISBN 9781118818152
   (Adobe PDF) | ISBN 9781118818169 (ePub) | ISBN 9781118818176 (pbk.)
Subjects: | MESH: Electrocardiography | Handbook
Classification: LCC RC683.5.E5 (ebook) | LCC RC683.5.E5 (print) | NLM WG 39 | DDC 616.1/207547–dc23
LC record available at https://lccn.loc.gov/2018060335

Cover Design: Wiley
Cover Image: © T VECTOR ICONS/ Shutterstock

Set in 9.25/12.5pt Helvetica Neue by SPi Global, Pondicherry, India

Printed in Great Britain by TJ International Ltd, Padstow, Cornwall

10 9 8 7 6 5 4 3 2 1

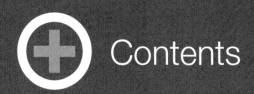

Contents

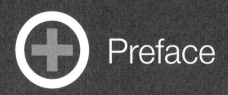

Preface

An electrocardiogram (ECG) is a recording of electrical waveforms produced by the electrical activity of the heart. ECG monitoring is probably one of the most valuable diagnostic tools in modern medicine. It is essential if cardiac arrhythmias are to be identified. It can help with diagnosis and can alert clinical staff to changes in the patient's condition. ECG monitoring must be meticulously undertaken. Potential consequences of poor technique include misinterpretation of cardiac arrhythmias, mistaken diagnosis, wasted investigations, and mismanagement of the patient.

The purpose of this guide is to provide a structured approach to the recognition and treatment of cardiac arrhythmias as well as providing guidance to the interpretation of the 12 lead ECG.

Philip Jevon
Jayant Gupta

About the companion website

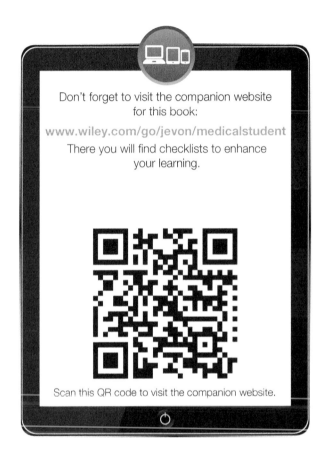

Don't forget to visit the companion website for this book:

www.wiley.com/go/jevon/medicalstudent

There you will find checklists to enhance your learning.

Scan this QR code to visit the companion website.

Introduction to ECG monitoring

1

Conduction system of the heart (figure 1.1)

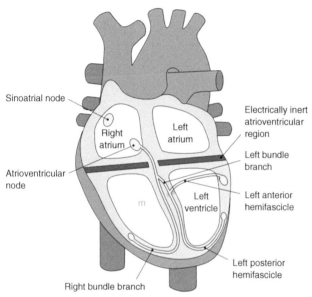

Figure 1.1 Conduction system of the heart.

PQRST complex (figure 1.2)

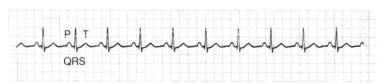

Figure 1.2 PQRST complex.

Medical Student Survival Skills: ECG, First Edition. Philip Jevon and Jayant Gupta.
© 2020 John Wiley & Sons Ltd. Published 2020 by John Wiley & Sons Ltd.
Companion website: www.wiley.com/go/jevon/medicalstudent

- *P wave*: atrial depolarisation
- *PR interval*: atrial depolarisation and the impulse delay in the atrioventricular (AV) node prior to ventricular depolarisation
- *QRS complex*: ventricular depolarisation
- *T wave*: ventricular repolarisation

Sinus rhythm (figure 1.3)

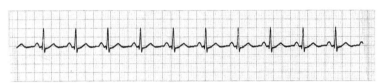

Figure 1.3 Sinus rhythm.

- Normal rhythm of the heart
- Impulse originates in the sinoatrial (SA) node (i.e. 'sinus'), regular rate of 60–100 beats per minute (bpm)
- No abnormal conduction delays

Sinus rhythm: Identifying ECG features
- *Electrical activity*: present
- *QRS rate*: 60–100 bpm
- *QRS rhythm*: regular
- *QRS width*: normal width and morphology
- *P waves*: present and of constant morphology
- *Relationship between P waves and QRS complexes*: P waves associated to QRS complexes; PR interval normal and constant

NB Sinus rhythm can occasionally be seen in a cardiac arrest: pulseless electrical activity (PEA).

2 Principles of ECG monitoring

Indications

Indications for ECG monitoring include:

- Critical illness
- Acute coronary syndromes
- Cardiac arrhythmias

ECG monitoring: Three ECG cable system (figure 2.1)

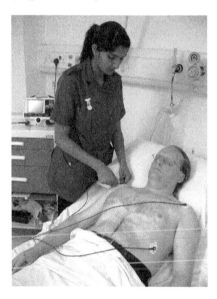

Figure 2.1 Three ECG cable system.

- Red ECG cable: below the right clavicle
- Yellow ECG cable: below the left clavicle
- Green ECG cable: left lower thorax/hip region

Medical Student Survival Skills: ECG, First Edition. Philip Jevon and Jayant Gupta.
© 2020 John Wiley & Sons Ltd. Published 2020 by John Wiley & Sons Ltd.
Companion website: www.wiley.com/go/jevon/medicalstudent

ECG monitoring: Five ECG cable system (figure 2.2)

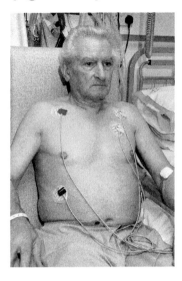

Figure 2.2 Five ECG cable system.

- RA (red ECG cable): below the right clavicle
- LA (yellow ECG cable): below the left clavicle
- RL (black ECG cable): right lower thorax/hip region
- LL (green ECG cable): left lower thorax/hip region
- V (white ECG cable): on the chest in the desired V position, usually V1 (4th intercostal space just right of the sternum)

ECG monitoring: Trouble shooting

'Flat line' trace
In a flat line trace (Figure 2.3) check if it is asystole. Check the patient, although asystole is rarely a straight line. It is usually a mechanical problem. Check:
- ECG monitoring lead selected on monitor, e.g. lead II
- ECG gain (effects size of complexes)
- Electrodes: in date, gel sponge moist, not dry?
- ECG cables: connected?

 NB Flat line ECG trace: always check the patient first – cardiac arrest?

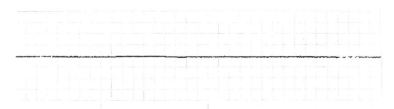

Figure 2.3 Flat line trace.

Wandering ECG baseline

A wandering ECG baseline (Figure 2.4) is usually caused by patient movement, particularly respirations. It may help to reposition the electrodes away from the lower ribs.

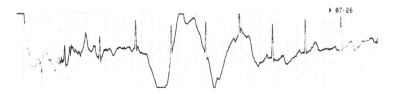

Figure 2.4 Wandering ECG baseline.

Electrical interference

This is usually caused by electrical interference from devices by the bedside, e.g. infusion pumps (Figure 2.5). Remove the source of the interference if possible.

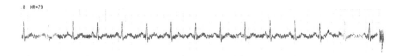

Figure 2.5 Electrical interference.

Insecure ECG electrode

A wandering ECG baseline, together with sudden breaks in the signal, suggests an insecure electrode (Figure 2.6). Ensure:
- Electrodes positioned correctly
- Skin interface is adequate, i.e. shave excess hair, dry skin if clammy
- ECG cables are not taught and tugging on electrodes

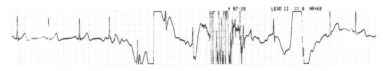

Figure 2.6 Insecure ECG electrode.

Small ECG complexes

The pathological causes of small ECG complexes (Figure 2.7) include pericardial effusion, obesity, and hypothyroidism. It may be a technical problem:

- Check ECG gain correctly set
- Select alternative ECG monitoring lead, e.g. lead I
- Try repositioning the electrodes

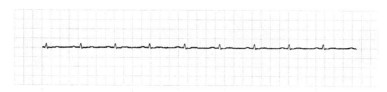

Figure 2.7 Small ECG complexes.

Unreliable heart rate display on monitor

Ensure there is an adequate ECG trace in order to avoid:

- Small ECG complexes: false-low heart rate may be displayed
- Large T waves, muscle movement and interference: may be mistaken for QRS complexes and false-high heart rate may be displayed

> ⚠️ **Common misinterpretations and pitfalls**
>
> The heart rate displayed on the ECG monitor can sometimes be grossly inaccurate: always check the patient.

Mechanisms of cardiac arrhythmias

- Altered automaticity leading to changes in the rate of impulse generation by the SA node
- Enhanced automaticity: causes include increased sympathetic activity, myocardial ischaemia, and drugs
- Re-entry self-perpetuating 'circus movement' of cardiac impulse

- Accessory pathways, e.g. bundle of Kent
- Triggered activity
- Reperfusion arrhythmias
- Conduction disturbances

OSCE Key Learning Points

ECG monitoring

✔ Explain procedure to patient

✔ Prepare skin prior to application of electrodes

✔ Select lead II on ECG monitor

✔ Interpret ECG following six stage approach

3 Six stage approach to ECG interpretation

- Electrical activity present?
- QRS rate?
- QRS rhythm: regular or irregular?
- QRS width: normal or broad?
- P waves present?
- Association between P and QRS?

(Source: Resuscitation Council [UK], 2018)

Electrical activity present?

If there is no electrical activity check the patient, gain control (ECG size), ECG leads, ECG electrodes, all electrical connections and defibrillator/cardiac monitor, ensuring it is switched on.

QRS rate?

- Count the number of large squares between adjacent QRS complexes and dividing it into 300, e.g. the QRS rate in Figure 1.3 is about 75 (300/4)
- If the QRS rhythm is obviously irregular count the number of QRS complexes in a defined number of seconds and then calculate the rate per minute. For example, if there are 10 QRS complexes in a 10 second strip, then the ventricular rate is 60 bpm (10 × 6)

Classify QRS rate:

- Normal: 60–100
- Bradycardia: <60
- Tachycardia: >100

 Common misinterpretations and pitfalls

A bradycardia is not always abnormal, e.g. it may be normal for an athlete or a desired effect of beta-blocker therapy.

Medical Student Survival Skills: ECG, First Edition. Philip Jevon and Jayant Gupta.
© 2020 John Wiley & Sons Ltd. Published 2020 by John Wiley & Sons Ltd.
Companion website: www.wiley.com/go/jevon/medicalstudent

QRS rhythm: Regular or irregular?

- Carefully compare RR intervals to ascertain if QRS rhythm is regular or irregular
- Plot two QRS complexes on a piece of paper, move this to other sections on the ECG rhythm strip and determine if the QRS marks are aligned

Irregular QRS rhythm: totally irregular, e.g. in atrial fibrillation, or cyclical pattern to the irregularity, e.g. extrasystoles, pauses, or dropped beats?

QRS width: Normal or broad?

- Measure width of QRS complex (normal width is <3 small squares or 0.12 seconds)

NB Broad QRS (3 small squares or 0.12 seconds or greater): the QRS rhythm may be ventricular or supraventricular (transmitted with aberrant conduction). A broad complex tachycardia is usually ventricular.

- Examine all QRS complexes: constant morphology?

P present?

Check if P waves are present: calculate the rate, regularity, and morphology

NB P waves should precede each QRS complex, and should be identical in shape and upright in lead II.

Relationship between P and QRS?

- Check if P waves and QRS complexes are associated
- Calculate PR interval (normal 3–5 small squares or 0.12–0.20 seconds); should be constant
- A shortened or prolonged PR interval is indicative of a conduction abnormality
- Constant PR interval: P and QRS complexes are probably associated
- Variable PR interval: may be due to AV block
- Complete dissociation between P and QRS complexes: may indicate third degree AV heart block.

OSCE Key Learning Points

ECG rhythm interpretation
- ✔ Electrical activity present (yes/no)
- ✔ QRS rate (normal, fast, slow)
- ✔ QRS rhythm (regular/irregular)
- ✔ QRS width (normal/broad)
- ✔ P waves present
- ✔ Relationship between P waves and QRS

④ Sinus tachycardia

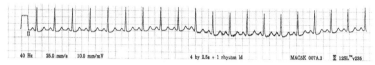

Figure 4.1 Sinus tachycardia.

- Sinus rhythm > 100 bpm (usually < 140 bpm)

Causes

Causes include:
- Shock
- Heart failure
- Anxiety
- Medications

Identifying ECG features

- *Electrical activity*: yes
- *QRS rate*: > 100 bpm, usually < 140 bpm
- *QRS rhythm*: regular.
- *QRS width*: normal and constant morphology
- *P waves*: present, may be merged into preceding T waves
- *Relationship between P waves and QRS complexes*: each P wave followed by a QRS, each QRS preceded by a P; PR interval normal and constant

Effects on patient

- Usually no symptoms, although the patient may be 'aware' of a fast bounding pulse

Treatment

- Identify and where appropriate treat the underlying cause
- Rarely: a beta-blocker such as atenolol to slow the heart (caution), e.g. persistent tachycardia associated with myocardial infarction

 Common misinterpretations and pitfalls

In most cases, sinus tachycardia itself should not be treated: treatment should target the underlying cause (if necessary).

5 Sinus bradycardia

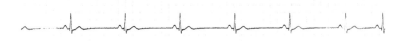

Figure 5.1 Sinus bradycardia.

- Sinus rhythm <60 bpm

Causes

Causes include:
- Acute myocardial infarction, particularly inferior myocardial infarction
- Raised intracranial pressure
- Medications, e.g. beta-blockers
- Vagal stimulation

Identifying ECG features

- *Electrical activity*: present
- *QRS rate*: <60 bpm
- *QRS rhythm*: regular
- *QRS width*: normal width and constant morphology
- *P waves*: present, constant morphology
- *Relationship between P waves and QRS complexes*: P followed by a QRS and each QRS preceded by a P; PR interval normal and constant

Medical Student Survival Skills: ECG, First Edition. Philip Jevon and Jayant Gupta.
© 2020 John Wiley & Sons Ltd. Published 2020 by John Wiley & Sons Ltd.
Companion website: www.wiley.com/go/jevon/medicalstudent

Effects on patient

- May lead to a fall in cardiac output: adverse signs could include hypotension, chest pain, lightheadiness, dizziness, nausea, syncope, and palor
- Note that there are normal physiological findings in some patients, e.g. athletes

Treatment

- Treatment is indicated only if adverse signs are present and/or there is a risk of asystole (see Resuscitation Council [UK] bradycardia algorithm in Appendix A)

6 Sinus arrhythmia

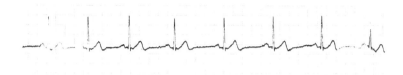

Figure 6.1 Sinus arrhythmia.

- A variation of sinus rhythm characterised by alternate periods of slow and more rapid SA node discharge
- QRS rhythm slightly irregular (normal finding usually associated with the phases of respiration, increasing with inspiration and decreasing with expiration)
- Variation of RR intervals due to a vagally mediated response to increased venous return to the heart during inspiration
- Common finding in younger persons

Identifying ECG features

- *Electrical activity*: present
- *QRS rate*: 60–100 bpm
- *QRS rhythm*: slightly irregular
- *QRS width*: normal and constant morphology
- *P waves*: present and constant morphology
- *Relationship between P waves and QRS complexes*: each P followed by a QRS and each QRS preceded by a P; PR interval normal and constant

Medical Student Survival Skills: ECG, First Edition. Philip Jevon and Jayant Gupta.
© 2020 John Wiley & Sons Ltd. Published 2020 by John Wiley & Sons Ltd.
Companion website: www.wiley.com/go/jevon/medicalstudent

Effects on patient

- Patient asymptomatic

Treatment

- No treatment required

7 Atrial ectopic beats

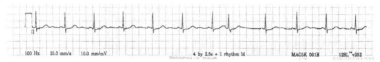

Figure 7.1 Atrial ectopics (atrial premature beats).

- Sometimes called atrial premature beats (APBs)
- Caused by a focus in the atria firing earlier in the cardiac cycle than the next timed beat would be expected
- May herald the onset of atrial fibrillation, atrial flutter, or atrial tachycardia
- P wave polarity and morphology will differ to P waves associated with sinus rhythm

Causes

Cause include:
- Cardiac stimulants, e.g. tobacco, caffeine, and alcohol
- Ischaemic heart disease
- Chronic obstructive pulmonary disease (CPOD)
- Electrolyte imbalance

Identifying ECG features

- *Electrical activity*: present
- *QRS rate*: usually normal, though dependent upon underlying rhythm and frequency of APBs
- *QRS rhythm*: slightly irregular owing to presence of APBs
- *QRS width*: usually normal and constant morphology; the prematurity of the APB may occasionally result in the impulse being conducted to the ventricles with bundle branch block – QRS morphology will then differ

Medical Student Survival Skills: ECG, First Edition. Philip Jevon and Jayant Gupta.
© 2020 John Wiley & Sons Ltd. Published 2020 by John Wiley & Sons Ltd.
Companion website: www.wiley.com/go/jevon/medicalstudent

- *P waves*: present; those associated with APBs will be of different morphology from sinus P waves and may be superimposed on the preceding T waves
- *Relationship between P waves and QRS complexes*: each P followed by a QRS and each QRS preceded by a P; PR interval may be marginally longer than in sinus rhythm

Effects on patient

- Usually asymptomatic

Treatment

- Atrial ectopics are benign and no treatment is necessary
- Attention to causes may be appropriate

 NB Atrial ectopics may be a precursor of atrial fibrillation.

8 Atrial tachycardia

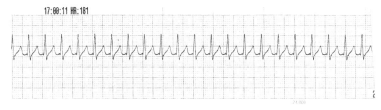

Figure 8.1 Atrial tachycardia.

- Ectopic focus in the atria rapidly depolarizing and overriding the normal pacemaker function of the SA node
- Often preceded by atrial ectopics (see Chapter 7)
- Characterised by a sudden onset and an abrupt end
- Atrial rate is normally between 150 and 200 bpm

Causes

Causes include:
- Ischaemic heart disease
- Rheumatic heart disease
- Cardiomyopathy

Identifying ECG features

- *Electrical activity*: present
- *QRS rate*: usually 150–200 bpm
- *QRS rhythm*: regular
- *QRS width*: normal width and morphology

Medical Student Survival Skills: ECG, First Edition. Philip Jevon and Jayant Gupta.
© 2020 John Wiley & Sons Ltd. Published 2020 by John Wiley & Sons Ltd.
Companion website: www.wiley.com/go/jevon/medicalstudent

- *P waves*: rate between 150 and 200 bpm, may not be visible, may be merged into preceding T waves; if visible, different morphology to sinus P waves
- *Relationship between P waves and QRS complexes*: difficult to ascertain relationship; PR interval often cannot be determined because P waves are not clearly distinguishable; if there is AV block, P waves may not be conducted to the ventricles (usually 2 : 1 AV block, i.e. every other P wave is blocked)

Effects on patient

- May be associated with palpitations and/or haemodynamic compromise due to the loss of effective atrial contractions and a rapid ventricular rate

Treatment

- ABCDE approach
- Follow narrow complex tachycardia algorithm (see Resuscitation Council [UK] tachycardia algorithm in Appendix B)

NB When associated with an accessory conduction pathway, e.g. bundle of Kent (Wolff–Parkinson–White syndrome – see Chapter 31), some anti-arrhythmic medications, e.g. verapamil and digoxin, are contraindicated.

9 Atrial flutter

(a)

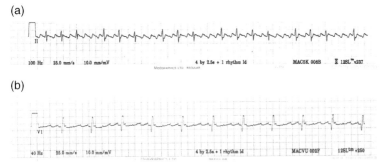

(b)

Figure 9.1 (a) Atrial flutter with varying AV block. (b) Atrial flutter with 4:1 AV block.

- Less common than atrial fibrillation
- Characterised by zigzagging baseline (sawtooth) flutter waves
- Often initiated by an atrial ectopic (see Chapter 7) and may degenerate into atrial fibrillation
- Atrial rate usually 300 bpm conducted to the ventricles (2:1 AV block); a regular tachycardia rate 150 bpm may be atrial flutter 2:1 AV block)

Causes

- Nearly always associated with significant cardiac disease, e.g. mitral valve disease
- Complicates 2–5% of acute myocardial infarctions
- Usually arises in the right atrium and often associated with diseases of the right side of the heart, e.g. chronic obstructive pulmonary disease (COPD), massive pulmonary embolism, and chronic congestive heart failure

Medical Student Survival Skills: ECG, First Edition. Philip Jevon and Jayant Gupta.
© 2020 John Wiley & Sons Ltd. Published 2020 by John Wiley & Sons Ltd.
Companion website: www.wiley.com/go/jevon/medicalstudent

Identifying ECG features

- *Electrical activity*: present
- *QRS rate*: dependent on the degree of AV block; usually 150 bpm
- *QRS rhythm*: regular or irregular (dependent on AV block)
- *QRS width*: normal width and constant morphology
- *P waves*: sawtooth flutter waves present, usually 300 min^{-1}; best seen in inferior leads and V1
- *Relationship between P waves and QRS complexes*: usually a degree of AV block is present, e.g. 2:1, 3:1, and 4:1 AV block; AV block may be variable

Effects on patient

- Patient may complain of rapid palpitations
- Sometimes atrial flutter is associated with haemodynamic compromise owing to the loss of effective atrial contractions and a rapid ventricular rate

Treatment

- ABCDE
- Consider pharmacology intervention as class 1 (e.g. sotolol, flecainide, or disopyramide) and class 3 (e.g. amiodarone) anti-arrhythmic drug therapy can terminate the tachycardia
- Seriously consider the early use of synchronised DC cardioversion where relatively low intensity shocks (e.g. 50 joules) often will effectively cardiovert and restore a sinus rhythm (must anticoagulate patients prior to DC cardioversion if flutter present more than 24–48 hrs. Offer longer term anticoagulation if flutter persists if CHADS2VASc score is 1 or more)
- Seek expert advice at an early stage

NB Carotid sinus massage (or IV adenosine) will often increase the level of AV block- QRS rate will fall and flutter waves may become more evident. It does not however terminate the arrhythmia as circus movement does not involve the AV node

⚠ Common misinterpretations and pitfalls

Atrial flutter with a 2 : 1 block is often mistaken as sinus tachycardia (QRS rate usually 150 bpm).

NB When associated with an accessory conduction pathway, e.g. bundle of Kent (Wolff–Parkinson–White syndrome – see Chapter 31), some anti-arrhythmic medications e.g. verapamil and digoxin, are contraindicated.

OSCE Key Learning Points

Treatment options for atrial flutter

✔ Control the ventricular rate or attempt to restore and maintain sinus rhythm

10 Atrial fibrillation

(a)

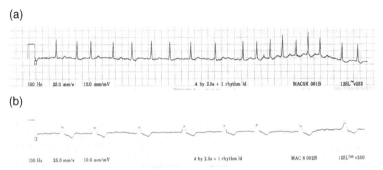

(b)

Figure 10.1 (a) Atrial fibrillation with a fast ventricular response. (b) Atrial fibrillation with a slow ventricular response.

- Atria discharge at a rate of 350–600 bpm: these impulses bombard the AV junction and are intermittently conducted to the ventricles resulting in the characteristic totally irregular QRS rhythm
- Ventricular rate will depend on the degree of AV conduction
- Usually triggered by an atrial ectopic; can be paroxysmal, persistent, or permanent (see Chapter 7)
- Prevalence increases with age; approximately 5% of individuals >69 years and 8% aged >80 years will experience it
- 15–25% of all strokes are associated with atrial fibrillation
- Box 10.1 lists the types of atrial fibrillation

Causes

Causes of atrial fibrillation include:
- Valvular heart disease
- Ischaemic heart disease
- Thyrotoxicosis
- Pulmonary disease

Medical Student Survival Skills: ECG, First Edition. Philip Jevon and Jayant Gupta.
© 2020 John Wiley & Sons Ltd. Published 2020 by John Wiley & Sons Ltd.
Companion website: www.wiley.com/go/jevon/medicalstudent

> ## Box 10.1 Classification of atrial fibrillation
>
> - *First detected atrial fibrillation*: newly diagnosed, the cause will need to be identified
> - *Recurrent atrial fibrillation*: patients who have experienced two or more episodes of atrial fibrillation; categorized as either paroxysmal (ending <7 days) or chronic (lasting >7 days). The patient's history is important to determine the appropriate category
> - *Lone atrial fibrillation*: a cardiopulmonary cause cannot be identified
>
> (Source: Fuster et al. 2006)

Identifying ECG features

- *Electrical activity*: present
- *QRS rate*: may be slow, normal or rapid
- *QRS rhythm*: totally irregular (regular if third degree AV block present)
- *QRS width*: usually normal width and constant morphology
- *P waves*: not present; irregular baseline owing to fibrillation waves
- *Relationship between P waves and QRS complexes*: not applicable (no P waves present)

Effects on patient

- Can be asymptomatic
- Loss of 'atrial kick' (atrial contraction) can result in a decrease in cardiac output by 20–30%; this, together with a rapid ventricular response, can lead to a fall in cardiac output of up to 50%
- Heart failure may develop, particularly if the patient has coexistent valvular heart disease or impaired left ventricular function
- Symptoms may include palpitations, weakness, shortness of breath, chest pain, feeling faint, and syncope
- If atrial fibrillation persists >48 hours, stasis of blood in the fibrillating atria can lead to clot formation, i.e. increased risk of systemic thromboembolism

 NB Patients with atrial fibrillation should be assessed for their risk of stroke and the need for thromboprophylaxis.

Treatment

- ABCDE
- Follow tachycardia algorithm (see Resuscitation Council [UK] tachycardia algorithm in Appendix B)
- Take into account clinical setting in which atrial fibrillation occurs; any remediable factors should be addressed if possible
- Treatment aimed at:
  - Slowing down the ventricular response
  - Converting it to sinus rhythm (if possible)
  - Reducing the frequency and haemodynamic effects of subsequent atrial
  - Fibrillation or preventing further episodes
  - Correcting any electrolyte imbalances

NB When associated with an accessory conduction pathway, e.g. bundle of Kent (Wolff–Parkinson–White syndrome – see Chapter 31), some anti-arrhythmic medications, e.g. verapamil and digoxin, are contraindicated.

OSCE Key Learning Points

Treatment options for atrial fibrillation

✔ Control the ventricular rate or attempt to restore and maintain sinus rhythm

11 AV junctional ectopics

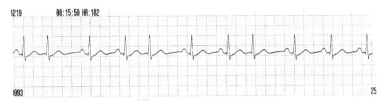

1219	08:15:59 HR:182
1993	25

Figure 11.1 AV junction ectopics.

- Caused by a focus in the AV junction depolorising earlier in the cardiac cycle than the next timed beat would be expected
- Less common than atrial and ventricular ectopics
- Can be a normal finding

Causes

Causes include:

- Cardiac stimulants, e.g. tobacco, caffeine, and alcohol
- Ischaemic heart disease
- Electrolyte imbalance

Identifying ECG features

- *Electrical activity*: present
- *QRS rate*: determined by the underlying rhythm
- *QRS rhythm*: slightly irregular owing to junctional premature beats
- *QRS width*: usually normal width and same morphology as the QRS complexes associated with sinus beats; however, the prematurity of the beat may result in the impulse being conducted to the ventricles with aberration; junctional ectopics occur before the next anticipated sinus beat

Medical Student Survival Skills: ECG, First Edition. Philip Jevon and Jayant Gupta.
© 2020 John Wiley & Sons Ltd. Published 2020 by John Wiley & Sons Ltd.
Companion website: www.wiley.com/go/jevon/medicalstudent

- *P waves*: usually absent; if present they will be of different morphology from those associated with sinus beats, will usually be of opposite polarity to the QRS complexes (upright in V1 or inverted in lead II) and will be located immediately prior to or following the QRS complex
- *Relationship between P waves and QRS complexes*: if P waves are present they occur immediately prior to or following the QRS complexes; if measurable, the PR interval is short

Effects on patient

- Patient is usually asymptomatic

Treatment

- Treatment is not usually required
- Any electrolyte imbalances should be corrected

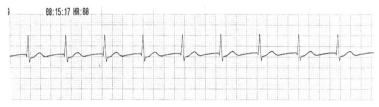

Figure 12.1 Junctional escape rhythm.

- Junctional escape rhythm is said to be present when there are six or more consecutive junctional escape beats
- This is not a primary diagnosis, rather a symptom of an underlying primary disturbance (SA node malfunction) to which it is secondary
- Inherent rate of AV junction is 40–60 bpm

Causes

- SA node failure (or malfunction) to initiate impulse

Identifying ECG features

- *Electrical activity*: present
- *QRS rate*: usually 40–60 bpm
- *QRS rhythm*: usually regular
- *QRS width*: usually normal width and same configuration as the QRS complexes associated with sinus beats
- *P waves*: usually absent; if present, are of different morphology from those associated with sinus beats, are of opposite polarity to the QRS complexes (upright in V1 or inverted in lead II) and occur immediately prior to or following the QRS complex

Medical Student Survival Skills: ECG, First Edition. Philip Jevon and Jayant Gupta.
© 2020 John Wiley & Sons Ltd. Published 2020 by John Wiley & Sons Ltd.
Companion website: www.wiley.com/go/jevon/medicalstudent

- *Relationship between P waves and QRS complexes*: if P waves are present they occur immediately prior to or following the QRS complexes; if measurable, the PR interval is short

Effects on patient

- If the rhythm is sustained, patient may become haemodynamically compromised, as loss of 'atrial kick' will contribute to the fall in cardiac output

Treatment

- Junctional escape rhythm itself does not require treatment and should not be suppressed by drugs
- Treatment is aimed at stimulating a higher pacemaker, e.g. atropine; pacing may be required
- Cause of SA node failure should be sought, e.g. medications, myocardial ischaemia/infarction. Any electrolyte imbalances should be corrected

NB Junctional escape rhythm: treatment aimed at speeding up SA node.

13 Junctional tachycardia

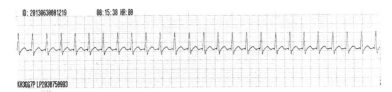

ID: 20130630081219   08:15:38 HR:80

KH3GG7P LP2830750993

Figure 13.1 Junctional tachycardia.

- Characterised by sudden onset and abrupt ending
- Regular rhythm typically a rate of 180–200 bpm
- Sometimes still referred to as supraventricular tachycardia (SVT)

Causes

Causes include:
- Ischaemic heart disease
- AV junctional disease

Identifying ECG Features

- *Electrical activity*: present
- *QRS rate*: usually 180–200 bpm
- *QRS rhythm*: usually regular
- *QRS width*: usually normal width and same morphology as the QRS complexes associated with sinus beats (unless aberrant conduction is present)
- *P waves*: usually not visible
- *Relationship between P waves and QRS complexes*: P waves usually not visible

Medical Student Survival Skills: ECG, First Edition. Philip Jevon and Jayant Gupta.
© 2020 John Wiley & Sons Ltd. Published 2020 by John Wiley & Sons Ltd.
Companion website: www.wiley.com/go/jevon/medicalstudent

Effects on patient

- Most will complain of palpitations
- Patient may become haemodynamically compromised. This is influenced by the rate, duration of the episode, and underlying cardiac disease

Treatment

- ABCDE
- Follow the tachycardia algorithm (see Resuscitation Council [UK] tachycardia algorithm in Appendix B)
- Vagal manoeuvres may slow or terminate junctional tachycardia
- Adenosine is usually first drug of choice
- If the patient is severely compromised and adverse signs are present or if other treatments fail, synchronised electrical cardioversion is usually undertaken
- Long-term treatment may include radiofrequency ablation
- Any electrolyte imbalances should be corrected

 NB Junctional tachycardia is sometimes referred to as SVT (supraventricular tachycardia).

⑭ Ventricular ectopics

- Ventricular ectopics (VEs) (ventricular premature beats) are caused by an ectopic focus in the ventricles
- Most ventricular ectopics are wide (0.12 seconds or 3 small squares or more) and bizarre in shape (this is caused by depolarisation across the ventricle walls, which increases the time for contraction to occur, as opposed to the normal His–Purkinje systems)
- Generally, an ectopic originating in the left ventricle has a right bundle branch block appearance (positive in V1), and one originating in the right ventricle has a left bundle branch block appearance (negative in V1)
- A full compensatory pause will usually follow – the term 'compensatory pause' is so called because the cycle following the ventricular ectopic compensates for its prematurity and the sinus rhythm then resumes on schedule

Ventricular ectopic terminology

- *Uniform or unifocal VEs*: VEs of the same morphology (Figure 14.1)
- *Multiform*: two or more VEs of distinctly different morphology (Figure 14.2)
- *R on T ventricular premature beat (VPB)*: a VE which 'lands' on the T wave
- *Ventricular bigeminy*: a VE after every sinus beat (Figure 14.3)
- *Ventricular trigeminy*: a VE after every two sinus beats (Figure 14.4)
- *Couplets*: pairs of VEs (Figure 14.5)
- *Salvos*: three or more consecutive VEs (Figure 14.6)

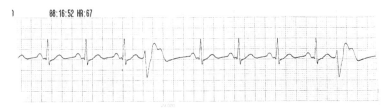

Figure 14.1 Unilateral ventricular premature beats.

Medical Student Survival Skills: ECG, First Edition. Philip Jevon and Jayant Gupta.
© 2020 John Wiley & Sons Ltd. Published 2020 by John Wiley & Sons Ltd.
Companion website: www.wiley.com/go/jevon/medicalstudent

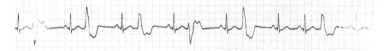

Figure 14.2 Multifocal ventricular premature beats.

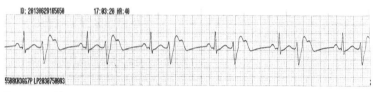

Figure 14.3 Ventricular bigeminy.

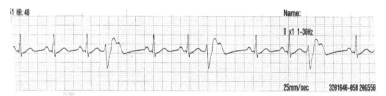

Figure 14.4 Ventricular trigeminy.

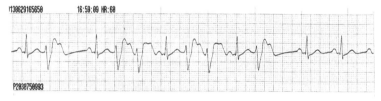

Figure 14.5 Salvos of ventricular premature beats.

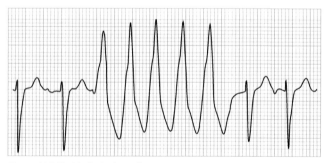

Figure 14.6 Ventricular tachycardia.

Causes

Causes include:

- Ischaemic heart disease
- Acute myocardial infarction
- Electrolyte imbalances
- Heart failure

Identifying ECG features

- *Electrical activity*: present
- *QRS rate*: determined by the underlying rhythm
- *QRS rhythm*: irregular due to presence of ectopics
- *QRS width*: the VE will be wide (0.12 seconds or 3 small squares or more), bizarre with changing amplitude, morphology, and deflection; morphology differs from that of the QRS complexes associated with the underlying rhythm; the ST segment usually slopes in a direction opposite to the QRS deflection; they occur before the next anticipated sinus beat and are usually followed by a compensatory pause
- *P waves*: usually none are visible (if visible, situated on the T wave due to retrograde conduction)
- *Relationship between P waves and QRS complexes*: usually not possible to determine the relationship between P waves and VEs

Effects on patient

- The patient is usually aware of the premature beat itself, of the subsequent pause often described as a missed beat, or of a stronger post-ectopic beat
- More noticeable at night when the patient is in a left lateral position
- Patient may be asymptomatic
- Can be associated with a significant fall in stroke volume and are often not pulse-producing; frequent ventricular ectopics can therefore have significant haemodynamic effects on the patient

Treatment

- Anti-arrhythmic therapy to suppress ventricular ectopics is no longer recommended
- When associated with acute myocardial infarction: adequate pain relief and effective treatment of heart failure
- Correction of any electrolyte imbalance

15 Idioventricular rhythm

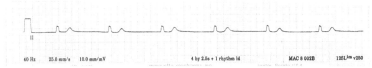

40 Hz	25.0 mm/s	10.0 mm/mV	4 by 2.5s + 1 rhythm ld	MAC 8 002B	12SL^{tm} v250

Figure 15.1 Idioventricular rhythm.

- Series of five or more consecutive ventricular escape beats
- Can occur if all potential pacemakers above the ventricles fail to initiate impulses, if the underlying rhythm is slower than the intrinsic ventricular rhythm, or if there is third degree (complete) AV block
- Not a primary diagnosis, rather a symptom of an underlying primary disturbance to which it is secondary

Causes

Causes include:
- Acute myocardial infarction
- Reperfusion following reperfusion therapy
- Drugs
- Electrolyte imbalance

Identifying ECG features

- *Electrical activity*: present
- *QRS rate*: usually 20–40 bpm
- *QRS rhythm*: usually regular
- *QRS width*: usually wide (0.12 seconds or 3 small squares or more) and bizarre; ventricular premature beat (VPB) morphology differs from that of the QRS complexes associated with the underlying rhythm; ST segment

Medical Student Survival Skills: ECG, First Edition. Philip Jevon and Jayant Gupta.
© 2020 John Wiley & Sons Ltd. Published 2020 by John Wiley & Sons Ltd.
Companion website: www.wiley.com/go/jevon/medicalstudent

usually slopes in an opposite direction to the QRS deflection; usually starts after a pause in the underlying rhythm

- *P waves*: usually absent, though may be present if complete AV block exists
- *Relationship between P waves and QRS complexes*: AV dissociation if AV block is present

Effects on patient

- The patient may be haemodynamically compromised, particularly if the rhythm is sustained or slow. The loss of 'atrial kick' will contribute to the fall in cardiac output; however, it is rarely sustained

Treatment

- Not usually required
- If treatment is required (rhythm sustained and patient haemodynamically compromised) it will be aimed at stimulating a higher pacemaker, e.g. atropine to speed up the underlying rhythm
- It may be necessary to identify and treat the cause of SA node and AV junction failure

16 Ventricular tachycardia

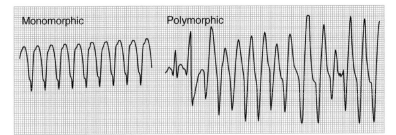

Figure 16.1 Ventricular tachycardia.

- Ventricular tachycardia (VT) is diagnosed if there are three or more successive ventricular ectopics at a rate of >120 minutes; it is classed as sustained VT if it lasts for more than 30 seconds and unsustained VT if it lasts for less than 30 seconds
- QRS complexes are wide (0.12 seconds or 3 small squares or more) and bizarre. Monomorphic VT is when the QRS complexes are of constant shape. Polymorphic VT is when the QRS morphology changes ('torsades de points') (Figure 16.1) (see Chapter 17)
- If atria continue to depolarise independently of the ventricle, i.e. AV dissociation, then some P waves may be visible (positive in lead II); sometimes this independent atrial activity can lead to fusion and capture beats, the presence of which are hallmarks of VT
- Most broad complex tachycardias are ventricular in origin, i.e. VT. Occasionally a supraventricular tachycardia can be conducted with bundle branch block resulting in a broad complex tachycardia. Twelve lead ECGs should be recorded whenever possible to help confirm diagnosis

Medical Student Survival Skills: ECG, First Edition. Philip Jevon and Jayant Gupta.
© 2020 John Wiley & Sons Ltd. Published 2020 by John Wiley & Sons Ltd.
Companion website: www.wiley.com/go/jevon/medicalstudent

Causes

Causes include

- Ischaemic heart disease
- Myocardial infarction
- Cardiomyopathy
- Electrolyte imbalance

Identifying ECG features

- *Electrical activity*: present
- *QRS rate*: usually 150–200 bpm
- *QRS rhythm*: regular or irregular
- *QRS width*: wide (0.12 seconds or 3 small squares or more) and bizarre; ventricular premature beat (VPB) morphology differs from the QRS complexes associated with the underlying rhythm; ST segment usually slopes in a direction opposite to the QRS deflection
- *P waves*: may be present
- *Relationship between P waves and QRS complexes*: if P waves are visible, AV dissociation is often present

Fusion and capture beats

- Fusion beat (Figure 16.2): when an impulse from the SA node travelling antegradely meets an impulse from the ventricles travelling retrogradely. The ventricles are therefore depolarised partly by the impulse being conducted through the His–Purkinje system and partly by the impulse arising in the ventricle. The resultant QRS complex partly resembles a normal complex and partly resembles a VPB complex
- Capture beat (Figure 16.3): when an impulse from the SA node is conducted to the ventricles resulting in a P wave followed by a normal QRS complex

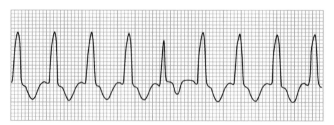

Figure 16.2 Fusion beat.

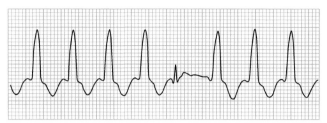

Figure 16.3 Capture beat.

Effects on patient

- Ventricular tachycardia is a serious cardiac arrhythmia. The patient will often be haemodynamically compromised. In some patients cardiac output will be lost
- It can degenerate into ventricular fibrillation (see Chapter 22)

 NB Sustained ventricular tachycardia can lead to loss in cardiac output and cardiac arrest.

Treatment

- Patient pulseless: immediate defibrillation – follow Resuscitation Council (UK) advanced life support (ALS) algorithm (see Appendix C)
- Patient has a pulse: ABCDE and follow the Resuscitation Council (UK) tachycardia algorithm (see Appendix B)
- Chemical cardioversion is usually required for sustain VT
- Electrical cardioversion may be indicated (see Appendix E)
- Any electrolyte imbalances should be corrected if possible

 Uncommon presentations

Board complex tachycardia can occasionally be a supraventricular tachycardia conducted with aberration, i.e. not VT.

17 Torsades de pointes

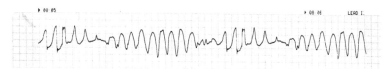

Figure 17.1 Torsades de pointes.

- Polymorphic (changing shape of the QRS complex) ventricular tachycardia sometimes referred to as 'torsades de pointes'
- The French word 'torsades' refers to an ornamental motif imitating twisted hairs or threads as seen on classical architectural columns, and 'pointes' refers to points or peaks
- Cardiac axis rotates over a sequence of 5–20 beats, changing from one direction to another and then back again
- ECG: spiky QRS complexes rotating irregularly around the isoelectric line at a rate of 200–250 bpm

 NB The administration of anti-arrhythmic drugs (sometimes administered for monomorphic VT) may make the arrhythmia worse.

Causes

Torsades de points is usually associated with a prolonged QT interval, causes of which include:
- Anti-arrhythmic drugs
- Bradycardia due to sick sinus syndrome or AV block
- Congenital prolongation of the QT interval, e.g. Romano–Ward syndrome
- Electrolyte imbalance, e.g. hypokalaemia and hypomagnesaemia

Medical Student Survival Skills: ECG, First Edition. Philip Jevon and Jayant Gupta.
© 2020 John Wiley & Sons Ltd. Published 2020 by John Wiley & Sons Ltd.
Companion website: www.wiley.com/go/jevon/medicalstudent

Identifying ECG features

- *Electrical activity*: present
- *QRS rate*: usually 200–250 bpm
- *QRS rhythm*: irregular
- *QRS width*: wide (0.12 seconds or 3 small squares or more) and bizarre, with changing amplitude, polarity, morphology, and deflection
- *P waves*: unable to identify
- *Relationship between P waves and QRS complexes*: AV dissociation may be present

Effects on patient

- May become haemodynamically compromised
- Sometimes may degenerate into ventricular fibrillation and cardiac arrest

Treatment

- Effective treatment, i.e. prevention of recurrent episodes, involves attention to the presumed predisposing cause(s), e.g. stopping offending drug and correction of any electrolyte imbalances
- Overdrive pacing may be effective
- Measures to speed up the sinus rate may be effective in some situations

18 First degree AV block

(a)

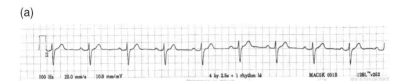

(b)

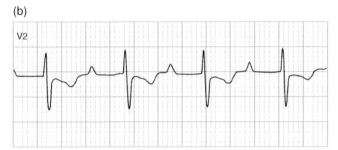

Figure 18.1 (a and b) First degree AV block.

- There is a delay (usually in AV junction) in the conduction of atrial impulses to the ventricles
- it is characterised by a prolonged but constant PR interval (>0.20 seconds or 5 small squares) (Figure 18.1), all the impulses are conducted to the ventricles and there are no missed beats
- It is usually benign
- If associated with acute myocardial infarction, close monitoring of the ECG is required because there may be a progression to a higher degree of AV block
- Sometimes it is a normal phenomenon: in young persons it is usually due to increased vagal tone and is benign

Medical Student Survival Skills: ECG, First Edition. Philip Jevon and Jayant Gupta.
© 2020 John Wiley & Sons Ltd. Published 2020 by John Wiley & Sons Ltd.
Companion website: www.wiley.com/go/jevon/medicalstudent

Causes

Causes include:
- Inferior myocardial infarction
- Ischaemic heart disease
- Electrolyte imbalance
- Medications, e.g. beta-blockers

Identifying ECG features

- *Electrical activity*: present
- *QRS rate*: usually normal
- *QRS rhythm*: usually regular
- *QRS width*: normal width and morphology
- *P waves*: present and constant morphology
- *Relationship between P waves and QRS complexes*: each P wave is followed by a QRS complex and each QRS complex is preceded by a P wave; PR interval is prolonged, i.e. >0.20 seconds or 5 small squares

Effects on patient

- The patient will be asymptomatic

Treatment

- Requires no specific treatment, although drugs that can prolong AV conduction, e.g. beta-blockers, will probably need to be avoided

19 Second degree AV block Mobitz type I (Wenckebach phenomenon)

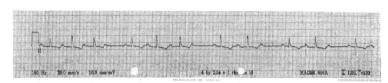

Figure 19.1 Second degree AV block Mobitz type I.

- There are two classifications of second degree AV block: Mobitz type I (Wenckebach phenomenon) and Mobitz type II (see Chapter 20) (both are named after Woldemar Mobitz, an early twentieth century German internist)
- Second degree AV block Mobitz type I (Wenckebach phenomenon – named after Karel Wenckebach, a Dutch anatomist) is the most common (90%) type of second degree AV block
- Intermittent failure of transmission of the atrial impulse to the ventricles
- Characterised by a progressive prolongation of the PR interval (the footprints of the Wenckeback phenomenon) until an impulse fails to be conducted to the ventricles, resulting in a dropped beat (QRS complex). This is then followed by a conducted impulse, a shorter PR interval, and a repetition of the cycle
- The number of dropped beats is variable

Causes

Causes include:
- Inferior myocardial infarction
- Electrolyte imbalance

Medical Student Survival Skills: ECG, First Edition. Philip Jevon and Jayant Gupta.
© 2020 John Wiley & Sons Ltd. Published 2020 by John Wiley & Sons Ltd.
Companion website: www.wiley.com/go/jevon/medicalstudent

- Drugs that suppress AV conduction, e.g. beta-blockers, digoxin, and calcium channel blockers
- Increased vagal tone during sleep

Identifying ECG features

- *Electrical activity*: present
- *QRS rate*: depending on the number of dropped beats, may be bradycardic
- *QRS rhythm*: usually irregular (unless 2 : 1 conduction)
- *QRS width*: usually normal width and morphology
- *P waves*: present and constant morphology, PP interval remains constant
- *Relationship between P waves and QRS complexes*: not every P wave is followed by a QRS, but every QRS complex is preceded by a P wave; PR interval progressively lengthens until a QRS complex is dropped; RR interval progressively shortens

Effects on patient

- Usually asymptomatic
- If the ventricular rate is slow, then the patient could become haemodynamically compromised (rare)

Treatment

- Treatment not usually required
- Avoid drugs that may potentiate the AV block, e.g. beta-blockers
- Follow the Resuscitation Council (UK) bradycardia algorithm (see Appendix A) if necessary

20 Second degree AV block Mobitz type II

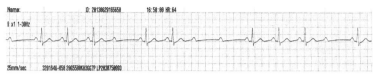

Figure 20.1 Second degree AV block Mobitz type II.

- There are two classifications of second degree AV block (see Chapter 19)
- There is intermittent failure of transmission of the atrial impulse to the ventricles
- The number of dropped beats is variable
- It is less common than second degree AV block type I, but its implications are significantly more serious
- Block is usually at the level of the bundle branches, commonly resulting in a wide QRS complex
- It can suddenly progress to third degree (complete) AV block (see Chapter 21) or even ventricular standstill (see Chapter 23)
- It is never a normal clinical finding

Causes

Causes include:
- Acute myocardial infarction, particularly anterior
- Drugs that suppress AV conduction, e.g. beta-blockers, digoxin, and calcium channel blockers

Identifying ECG features

- *Electrical activity*: present
- *QRS rate*: depends on the number of dropped beats; may be normal or bradycardic

Medical Student Survival Skills: ECG, First Edition. Philip Jevon and Jayant Gupta.
© 2020 John Wiley & Sons Ltd. Published 2020 by John Wiley & Sons Ltd.
Companion website: www.wiley.com/go/jevon/medicalstudent

- *QRS rhythm*: usually irregular due to dropped beats (unless 2 : 1 conduction)
- *QRS width*: usually wide (0.12 seconds or 3 small squares or more) with bundle branch block pattern; may be normal width and morphology
- *P waves*: present and constant morphology
- *Relationship between P waves and QRS complexes*: not every P wave is followed by a QRS complex (dropped beats); every QRS complex is preceded by a P wave; PR interval is constant, but may be prolonged

Effects on patient

- The patient is often haemodynamically compromised
- Progression to ventricular standstill and cardiac arrest is not uncommon

Treatment

- Prophylactic temporary pacing is usually required

 Uncommon presentations

Second degree AV block Mobitz type II is rare but always serious: expert help should always be sought.

21 Third degree (complete) AV block

(a)

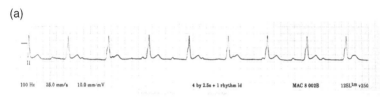

(b)

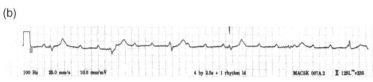

Figure 21.1 Third degree (complete) AV block with a ventricular rate of (a) 50 bpm and (b) 35 bpm.

- Third degree (complete) AV block is where there is total failure of conduction between the atria and ventricle
- It is characterised by AV dissociation – the P waves bear no relation to the QRS complexes and there is total independence of atrial and ventricular contractions
- It can be an acute phenomenon usually associated with a myocardial infarction or may be chronic, usually caused by fibrosis of the bundle of His
- When associated with an acute inferior myocardial infarction, it is normally caused by ischaemia or necrosis of the AV junction, and develops slowly, being often preceded by first degree and then second degree AV block Mobitz type 1 (Wenckebach). Generally well tolerated and the QRS complex may be narrow, signifying a junctional escape rhythm (see Chapter 12) which is usually reliable and of an adequate rate.
- When associated with anterior myocardial infarction, it is normally caused by extensive necrosis of the septum, with damage to both the left and right bundle branches; it is frequently a sudden event, especially in patients who

Medical Student Survival Skills: ECG, First Edition. Philip Jevon and Jayant Gupta.
© 2020 John Wiley & Sons Ltd. Published 2020 by John Wiley & Sons Ltd.
Companion website: www.wiley.com/go/jevon/medicalstudent

develop second degree AV block Mobitz type II or left bundle branch block. The QRS complex is wide, signifying a ventricular escape rhythm, unreliable and slow

- It is a common clinical finding in elderly patients admitted with a history of weakness, fatigue, 'off legs', syncope, etc. (typically in the preceding few weeks) – routine 12 lead ECG confirms diagnosis (a permanent pacemaker is the usual treatment)
- Rate and morphology of the escape rhythm is determined by the origin of the ventricular escape rhythm: if the pacemaker site is situated in the AV junction or proximal aspect of the bundle of His (more reliable), then the ventricular rate will be between 40 and 50 bpm (sometimes more) and the QRS width will be narrow; if the pacemaker site is in the distal His–Purkinje fibres or ventricular myocardium (less reliable), then the ventricular rate will be between 30 and 40 bpm (sometimes less) and the QRS width will be wide – sudden ventricular standstill and cardiac arrest is possible

Causes

Causes include:

- Acute myocardial infarction
- Fibrosis of bundle of His
- Endocarditis
- Drugs

Identifying ECG features

- *Electrical activity*: present
- *QRS rate*: dependent upon the site of the subsidiary pacemaker; 40–60 if junctional, 40 if ventricular
- *QRS rhythm*: regular
- *QRS width*: may be normal (if junctional pacemaker), otherwise wide (0.12 seconds or 3 small squares or more) with bundle branch block pattern (ventricular pacemaker)
- *P waves*: present and constant morphology, usually faster rate than the QRS complexes; absent if underlying rhythm is atrial fibrillation
- *Relationship between P waves and QRS complexes*: AV dissociation

Effects on patient

- Some patients will have an adequate escape rhythm that will maintain their blood pressure, while others will be compromised requiring urgent intervention
- Generally the effects on the patient will depend on the cause: when associated with an anterior myocardial infarction, the patient is haemodynamically compromised. The risk of ventricular standstill and sudden cardiac arrest is high. If associated with an inferior myocardial infarction the patient may be haemodynamically stable. If chronic, the patient may present with a history of blackouts or falls

 NB Complete AV block is sometimes seen in elderly patients who present with a history of lethargy, tiredness, and 'off legs'. It is not usually an acute problem: a permanent pacemaker is often required.

Treatment

- ABCDE approach
- Follow the Resuscitation Council (UK) bradycardia algorithm (see Appendix A)

22 Ventricular fibrillation

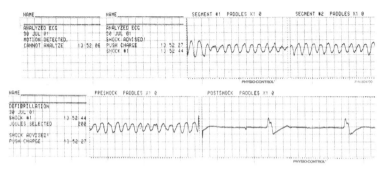

Figure 22.1 Ventricular fibrillation.

'The cardiac pump is thrown out of gear, and the last of its vital energy is dissipated in a violent and prolonged turmoil of fruitless activity in the ventricular walls…'

(Source: McWilliam 1889)

- Sudden cardiac arrest (SCA) causes approximately 700 000 out-of-hospital deaths in Europe each year; at least 40% are due to ventricular fibrillation
- In hospital, ventricular fibrillation is the presenting cardiac arrest arrhythmia in approximately 30% of arrests
- ECG features include a bizarre irregular waveform, apparently random in both amplitude and frequency, reflecting disorganised electrical activity in the myocardium
- Initially the amplitude of the waveform is coarse; this will rapidly deteriorate into asystole (see Chapter 24), reflecting the depletion of myocardial high-energy phosphate stores
- If there is electrical activity, but there are no recognisable complexes, the most likely diagnosis is ventricular fibrillation

Medical Student Survival Skills: ECG, First Edition. Philip Jevon and Jayant Gupta.
© 2020 John Wiley & Sons Ltd. Published 2020 by John Wiley & Sons Ltd.
Companion website: www.wiley.com/go/jevon/medicalstudent

Causes

Causes include:

- Ischaemic heart disease
- Heart failure
- Electrolyte imbalance
- Cardiomyopathy

Identifying ECG features

- *Electrical activity*: present
- *QRS rate*: no recognisable QRS complexes
- *QRS rhythm*: no recognisable QRS complexes
- *QRS width*: no recognisable QRS complexes
- *P waves*: none recognisable
- *Relationship between P waves and QRS complexes*: no recognisable P waves or QRS complexes present

Effects on patient

- Cardiac arrest

Treatment

- Rapid defibrillation is the definite treatment; give prompt cardiopulmonary resuscitation (CPR) while awaiting the defibrillator – follow the Resuscitation Council (UK) advanced life support (ALS) algorithm (see Appendix C)

OSCE Key Learning Points

Initial treatment of ventricular fibrillation

✔ Confirm cardiac arrest
✔ Alert the cardiac arrest team following local protocol (usually dial 2222)
✔ Rapid defibrillation
✔ CPR: particularly chest compressions

23 Ventricular standstill

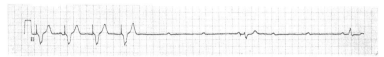

Figure 23.1 Ventricular standstill.

- Ventricular standstill is characterised by the presence of P waves and absent QRS complexes
- It is sometimes referred to as P wave asystole
- Sinus impulses are conducted to the ventricles, but the latter fail to respond to stimulation *or* sinus impulses are not conducted to the ventricles because of the presence of third degree (complete) AV block (see Chapter 21) and an idioventricular rhythm (see Chapter 15) fails to 'kick in'
- Can occur quite suddenly if the patient is already in second degree AV block Mobitz type II (see Chapter 20) or third degree (complete) AV block (see Chapter 21)

Causes

Causes of ventricular standstill include:
- Existing second degree AV block Mobitz type II or third degree (complete) AV block in the presence of acute anterior myocardial infarction
- Severe myocardial disease
- Drugs

Identifying ECG features

- *Electrical activity*: present
- *QRS rate*: no QRS complexes present
- *QRS rhythm*: no QRS complexes present

Medical Student Survival Skills: ECG, First Edition. Philip Jevon and Jayant Gupta.
© 2020 John Wiley & Sons Ltd. Published 2020 by John Wiley & Sons Ltd.
Companion website: www.wiley.com/go/jevon/medicalstudent

- *QRS width*: no QRS complexes present
- *P waves*: present
- *Relationship between P waves and QRS complexes*: no QRS complexes present

Effects on patient

- Cardiac arrest

Treatment

- Start cardiopulmonary resuscitation and follow the Resuscitation Council (UK) advanced life support (ALS) algorithm (see Appendix C)
- Emergency external pacing may be indicated. If capture is achieved and a pulse producing rhythm ensures, consider transvenous pacing

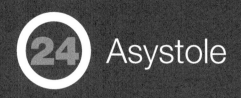

24 Asystole

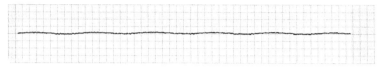

Figure 24.1 Asystole.

- Asystole is the presenting arrhythmia in approximately 25% of in-hospital cardiac arrests
- ECG – no electrical activity; P waves may be present
- Failure of sinus rhythm, under normal circumstances, will lead to the appearance of an escape rhythm maintained by a subsidiary pacemaker situated in either the AV junction (junctional rhythm) (see Chapter 12) or ventricular myocardium (idioventricular rhythm) (see Chapter 15)
- It is most important to ensure the ECG trace is accurate. Other causes of a 'flat line' ECG trace include incorrect lead and ECG gain settings, and disconnected ECG leads

Causes

Causes of asystole include:
- Myocardial disease
- Hypoxia
- Drugs
- Death

Identifying ECG features

- *Electrical activity*: no electrical activity present
- *QRS rate*: no electrical activity present
- *QRS rhythm*: no electrical activity present

Medical Student Survival Skills: ECG, First Edition. Philip Jevon and Jayant Gupta.
© 2020 John Wiley & Sons Ltd. Published 2020 by John Wiley & Sons Ltd.
Companion website: www.wiley.com/go/jevon/medicalstudent

- *QRS width*: no electrical activity present
- *P waves*: no electrical activity present
- *Relationship between P waves and QRS complexes*: no electrical activity present

Effects on patient

- Cardiac arrest

Treatment

- Start cardiopulmonary resuscitation (CPR) immediately – follow the Resuscitation Council (UK) advanced life support (ALS) algorithm (see Appendix C)

OSCE Key Learning Points

Initial treatment of asystole

✔ Confirm cardiac arrest

✔ Alert the cardiac arrest team following local protocol (usually dial 2222)

✔ CPR: particularly chest compressions

✔ Adrenaline 1 mg IV

---

25 Recording a 12 lead ECG

- An electrocardiograph is a machine that records the waveforms generated by the heart's electrical activity
- An electrocardiogram (ECG) is a record or display of a person's heartbeat produced by an electrocardiograph
- Care should taken to ensure accuracy and standardisation; poor technique can lead to misinterpretation of the ECG, mistaken diagnosis, wasted investigations, and mismanagement of the patient

Common indications

Common indications for recording a 12 lead ECG include:
- Chest pain
- Myocardial infarction
- Sometimes prior to a general anaesthetic
- Cardiac arrhythmias

Medical Student Survival Skills: ECG, First Edition. Philip Jevon and Jayant Gupta.
© 2020 John Wiley & Sons Ltd. Published 2020 by John Wiley & Sons Ltd.
Companion website: www.wiley.com/go/jevon/medicalstudent

Procedure

A suggested procedure for recording a standard 12 lead ECG is:

- Identify the patient
- Explain the procedure to the patient
- Assemble the equipment, ensuring that the ECG cables are not twisted as this can cause interference
- Ensure the environment is warm and the patient is as relaxed as possible. This will help produce a clear, stable trace without interference
- Ensure the patient is lying down in a comfortable position, ideally resting against a pillow at an angle of 45° with the head well supported (an identical patient position should be adopted as with previous 12 lead ECGs as this will help ensure standardisation). The inner aspects of the wrists should be close to, but not touching, the patient's waist
- Prepare the skin if necessary. If wet gel electrodes are used, shaving and abrading the skin is not required. If solid gel electrodes are used, clean/degrease and debrade the skin and shave if necessary
- Apply the electrodes and the limb leads:
    - Red to the inner right wrist
    - Yellow to the inner left wrist
    - Black to the inner right leg, just above the ankle
    - Green to the inner left leg, just above the ankle
- Apply the electrodes to the chest (Figure 25.1) and attach the chest leads:
    - V1 (white/red lead): 4th intercostal space, just to the right of sternum
    - V2 (white/yellow lead): 4th intercostal space, just to the left of sternum
    - V3 (white/green lead): midway between V2 and V4
    - V4 (white/brown lead): 5th intercostal space, mid-clavicular line
    - V5 (white/black lead): on anterior axillary line, on the same horizontal line as V4
    - V6 (white/violet lead): mid-axillary line, on the same horizontal line as V4 and V5
- Check the calibration signal on the ECG machine to ensure standardisation
- Ask the patient to lie still and breathe normally
- Print out the ECG following the manufacturer's recommendations
- Once an adequate 12 lead ECG has been recorded, disconnect the patient from the ECG machine and clear equipment away and clean as necessary following the manufacturer's recommendations. Sometimes electrodes are left on the patient if serial recordings are going to be required

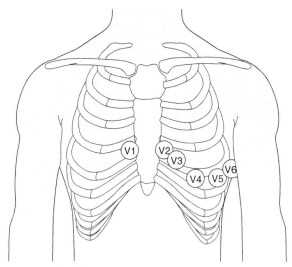

Figure 25.1 Position of chest electrodes.

- Ensure the ECG is correctly labelled. Report and store the ECG in the correct patient's notes following local procedures

Locating the intercostal spaces for the chest leads

Use the angle of Louis as a reference point for locating the 2nd intercostal space. The procedure is:
- Palpate the angle of Louis (sternal angle) – it is at the junction between the manubrium and the body of the sternum
- Slide the fingers towards the right side of the patient's chest and locate the 2nd rib, which is attached to the angle of Louis
- Slide the fingers down towards the patient's feet and locate the 2nd inter-costal space
- Slide the fingers further down to locate the 3rd and 4th ribs and the corresponding four intercostal spaces

 Common misinterpretations and pitfalls

Using the right clavicle as a reference to palpate the 1st intercostal space can lead to mistaking the space between the clavicle and the 1st rib as the 1st intercostal space.

Alternative chest lead placements

Alternative chest lead placements are sometimes indicated.

- *Right-sided*: inferior or posterior myocardial infarction, to ascertain whether there is right ventricular involvement (these patients may require careful management for hypotension and pain relief) and dextrocardia. The chest leads are labelled V3R to V6R and are in effect reflections of the left-sided chest leads V3–V6
- *Posterior*: particularly if there are reciprocal changes in V1–V2, suggesting posterior myocardial infarction. Chest leads are applied to the patient's back below the left scapula, corresponding to the same level as the 5th intercostal space, to view the posterior surface of the heart
- *Higher or more lateral on the chest*: if the clinical history is suggestive of myocardial infarction, but the ECG is inconclusive

Labelling the 12 lead ECG

- Labelling the 12 lead ECG should follow local protocols (often done electronically)
- All relevant information should be included, i.e. patient details (name, unit number, date of birth), date and time of recording, and ECG serial number together with any relevant information, e.g. if the patient was free from pain or complaining of chest pain during the recording, post reperfusion therapy
- The leads should be correctly labelled and deviations to the standard recording of a 12 lead ECG should be noted, e.g. right-sided chest leads, paper speed of $50\,\mathrm{mm\,s^{-1}}$, different patient position

Standardisation

- To help in the comparison of serial 12 lead ECGs, they should be recorded with the patient in the same position. If this is not possible, e.g. if the patient has orthopnoea, a note to this effect should be made because the electrical axis of the heart (main direct of current flow) can be altered which makes reviewing and comparing serial ECGs difficult
- Standard calibration is 1 mV vertical deflection on the ECG (Figure 25.2)
- Standard paper speed is $25\,\mathrm{mm\,s^{-1}}$

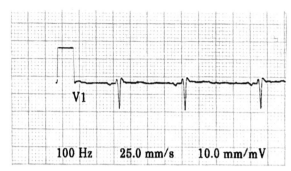

Figure 25.2 Standard calibration.

NB Any deviations to the standard procedure for the recording of a 12 lead ECG should be highlighted on the ECG. This will help to avoid possible misinterpretation and misdiagnosis.

26 What the standard 12 lead ECG records

- The heart generates electrical forces, which travel in multiple directions simultaneously. If the flow of current is recorded in several planes, a comprehensive view of this electrical activity can be obtained
- The standard 12 lead ECG records the electrical activity of the heart from 12 different viewpoints or leads ('leads' are viewpoints of the heart's electrical activity, they do not refer to the cables or wires that connect the patient to the monitor or ECG machine) by attaching 10 leads to the patient's limbs and chest

Limb leads

- If leads are attached to the patient's right arm, left arm, and left foot, the three major planes for detecting electrical activity can be recorded (a fourth lead, attached to the right leg serves as a neutral electrode and is not used for recording)
- A hypothetical triangle (Einthoven's triangle) is formed by these three axes, with the heart in the middle (Figure 26.1)
- These three different views of the heart are designated standard leads I, II, and III and each records the difference in electrical forces between the two lead sites, hence the term bipolar leads. This electrode placement also permits recording from three unipolar leads: aVR, aVL, and aVF

Chest leads

- The six chest leads view the heart in a horizontal plane from the front (anterior) and from the side (lateral)

Medical Student Survival Skills: ECG, First Edition. Philip Jevon and Jayant Gupta.
© 2020 John Wiley & Sons Ltd. Published 2020 by John Wiley & Sons Ltd.
Companion website: www.wiley.com/go/jevon/medicalstudent

Frontal plane

Bipolar leads

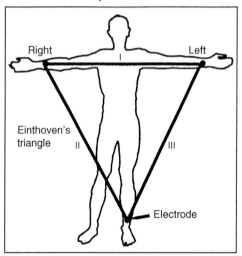

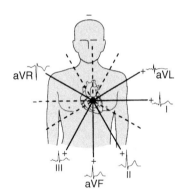

Figure 26.1 Einthoven's triangle.

Limb and chest leads and their relation to the surface of the heart

- *Inferior surface of the heart*: leads II, III, aVF (Figure 26.2)
- *Anterior surface of the heart*: leads V1, V2, V3, V4
- *Lateral surface of the heart*: leads I, aVL, V5, V6
- *Septum*: leads V2, V3

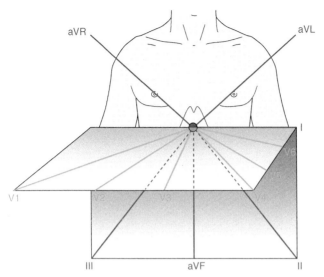

Figure 26.2 Limb and chest leads and their relation to the surface of the heart.

Configuration of the ECG waveform

- Electric current flows between two poles, a positive one and a negative one. An upward deflection will be recorded on the ECG when the current is flowing towards the positive pole; whereas a downward deflection will be recorded if the current is flowing away from the positive pole

- If an impulse is travelling towards a lead then the QRS complex in that lead will be predominantly positive, whereas if it is moving away from the lead it will be predominantly negative

- During depolarisation of the intraventricular septum, the impulse travels initially from left to right. The impulse then travels down the bundle branches and Purkinje fibres resulting in multidirectional and simultaneous ventricular depolarisation. In normal circumstances, the overall direction of depolarisation is towards the dominant mass of the left ventricle resulting in:
  - Small Q waves and tall R waves in leads facing the left ventricle, e.g. leads II, V5, V6
  - Small R waves and deep S waves in leads facing the right ventricle, e.g. V1, V2
  - R and S waves of equal size when the wave of depolarisation is at right angles to the lead, e.g. aVL

27 Interpretation of a 12 lead ECG

The following is a systematic approach to interpreting a 12 lead ECG:
- Patient and ECG details
- Calibration
- P waves
- PR interval
- QRS rate
- QRS rhythm
- QRS complexes
- T waves
- ST segment
- QT interval
- U waves
- Association between the P waves and QRS complexes
- Rhythm
- Electrical axis
- Previous ECGs

P waves

- Polarity: usually upright leads II, III, aVF
- Amplitude: not >0.3 mV (3 small squares)
- Width: not >0.11 seconds (2.75 small squares)
- Shape: round, not notched or pointed

- Amplitude: >0.3 mV: commonly due to atrial hypertrophy or dilation
- Duration: >0.11 seconds: commonly due to left atrial enlargement
- Inversion in leads II, III, and aVF: retrograde conduction
- Notching: left atrial enlargement (P mitrale)
- Peak complex: right atrial overload (P pulmonale)
- Diphasicity: left atrial enlargement

Medical Student Survival Skills: ECG, First Edition. Philip Jevon and Jayant Gupta.
© 2020 John Wiley & Sons Ltd. Published 2020 by John Wiley & Sons Ltd.
Companion website: www.wiley.com/go/jevon/medicalstudent

PR interval

- Normal: 0.12–0.20 seconds (3–5 small squares)
- PR interval >0.20 seconds (>5 small squares): first degree AV block
- PR interval <0.12 seconds (<3 small squares): AV junctional pacemaker or accessory pathway, e.g. bundle of Kent in Wolff–Parkinson–White syndrome

QRS rate

- Normal: 60–100 bpm
- QRS rate <60 bpm: bradycardia
- QRS rate >100 bpm: tachycardia

QRS rhythm

- Irregular QRS rhythm: many causes including sinus arrhythmia, atrial fibrillation, extrasystoles, and AV block

QRS complexes

- Q wave: if first deflection QRS is negative
- R wave: first positive deflection
- S wave: negative deflection following R wave
- R1: if second positive deflection
- S1: if second negative deflection
- Normal width: <0.12 seconds or 3 small squares; QRS width 0.12 seconds or 3 small squares or greater indicates abnormal intraventricular conduction (bundle branch block or ventricular arrhythmia)

Broad complex tachycardia is likely to be ventricular in origin if:
- R or qR (rabbit ear) in V1
- rS or QS in V6
- QRS complexes in V1–V6 are all either positive or negative
- Extreme axis deviation (−90° to ±180°) – positive aVR
- QRS complex >0.14 seconds or 3.5 small squares
- Presence of fusion beats and/or capture beats
- AV dissociation

Broad complex tachycardia is likely to be supraventricular in origin if:
- rsR morphology in V1
- qRs morphology in V6

- QRS morphology is the same as pre-existing bundle branch block pattern
- Right bundle branch block and the initial QRS deflection is identical to that with the normal rhythm

Total amplitude (voltage) of the QRS complex (above and below the isoelectric line) should be >0.5 mV (5 small squares) in the standard limb leads. An abnormally low voltage can be associated with pericardial effusion, myxoedema, and obesity.

QRS in V1: a dominant R wave of at least 0.5 mV (5 small squares) can be seen in right ventricular hypertrophy.

Tall R waves >2.5 mV (25 small squares) in leads V5 and V6 (deep S waves in V1) can be seen in left ventricular hypertrophy.

Q waves

Small narrow Q waves (<0.04 seconds or 1 small square wide and <0.2 mV or 2 small squares deep) are normal in leads facing the left ventricle, i.e. I, aVL, aVF, V5, and V6.

Wide (>0.04 seconds or 1 small square) and deep (>0.2 mV or 2 small squares) Q waves indicate previous myocardial infarction.

 NB Q waves in lead III can be a normal finding.

T waves

- *Polarity*: upright in leads I, II, and V3–V6, inverted in aVR; variable in the other leads. Inverted T waves can be associated with myocardial ischaemia, digoxin toxicity, or ventricular hypertrophy
- *Morphology*: normally slightly rounded and asymmetrical. Sharply pointed T waves suggest myocardial infarction or hyperkalaemia. Notched T waves may be associated with pericarditis. In myocardial ischaemia T waves can be tall, flattened, inverted, or biphasic. In left ventricular hypertrophy, T waves are inverted in the left ventricular leads, i.e. leads II, aVL, V5, and V6 in right ventricular hypertrophy, T waves are inverted in the right ventricular leads, i.e. V2 and V3
- *Height*: not >0.5 mV (5 small squares) in the limb leads or not >1.0 mV (10 small squares) in the chest leads

ST segment

- Isoelectric: normal
- Elevation >0.1 mV (1 small square) in limb leads and/or >0.2 mV (2 small squares) in the chest leads: usually indicates myocardial infarction
- Widespread concave ST segment elevation: characteristic of pericarditis
- ST segment elevation can be normal in healthy young black men
- Depression >0.5 mV (0.5 small squares): abnormal; horizontal depression of the ST segment and upright T wave usually indicates myocardial ischaemia
- ST segment down-sloping or sagging (particularly noticeable in leads II and III): suggests digoxin toxicity

QT interval

- Normal QT interval is usually less than half of the preceding RR interval; upper limit of normal is 0.40 seconds or 2 large squares
- Prolonged QT interval can lead to the development of tachyarrhythmias
- Causes of a prolonged QT interval: hereditary, drugs, hypothermia, and electrolyte abnormality

U waves

- Low voltage waves sometimes seen following the T waves
- Best seen in V3, share the same polarity as the T waves, and are usually more evident in hypokalaemia

Association between the P waves and QRS complexes

- Check if P waves and QRS complexes are associated
- Calculate PR interval (normal 3–5 small squares or 0.12–0.20 seconds); should be constant
- A shortened or prolonged PR interval is indicative of a conduction abnormality
- Constant PR interval: P and QRS complexes probably associated
- Variable PR interval: may be due to AV block
- Complete dissociation between P and QRS complexes: may indicate third degree AV heart block

Cardiac axis (figure 27.1)

(a)

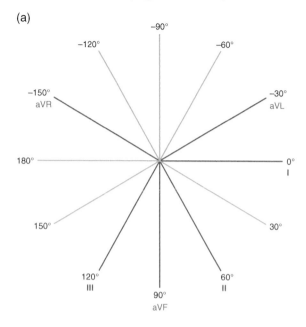

(b)

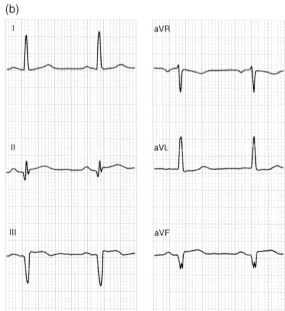

Figure 27.1 (a) Determining cardiac access using the hexaxial diagram. (b) Normal ECG axis.

- Normal axis is between 0° and +90°, left axis deviation is between 0° and −90°, and right axis deviation is between +90° and +180°
- Predominantly positive QRS in leads I and II: normal axis
- Predominantly positive QRS in lead I and predominantly negative QRS in lead II (the QRS complexes have 'left' each other): left axis deviation
- Predominantly negative QRS in lead I and predominantly positive QRS in lead II (QRS complexes are 'right' for each other): right axis deviation
- Causes of left axis deviation include left bundle branch block, left anterior fasicular block, and ventricular arrhythmias
- Causes of right axis deviation include right bundle branch block, left posterior fasicular block, and ventricular arrhythmias

Previous ECGs

- Compare with patient's previous ECGs; sequential ECGs in acute coronary syndrome can sometimes be particularly helpful in making a diagnosis

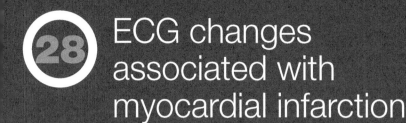

28 ECG changes associated with myocardial infarction

- >80% of patients with acute myocardial infarction present with an abnormal ECG
- <50% of patients initially present with typical and diagnostic ECG changes; sometimes the ECG may be normal or inconclusive
- Repeated ECGs may highlight ECG changes
- 10% of patients with a proved myocardial infarction (clinical history and raised troponin) fail to develop ST segment elevation or depression

Within minutes of myocardial infarction

- From being normal (Figure 28.1), T waves over the affected area become more pronounced, symmetrical, and pointed (Figure 28.2)
- These T waves, often referred to as 'hyperacute T waves', are more evident in the anterior leads and are more easily identified if an old 12 lead ECG is available for comparison
- These T wave changes are quickly followed by degrees of ST segment elevation (Figure 28.3), which is often seen in leads facing the affected area of the myocardium. It is caused by damaged, but not necrosed, myocardial tissue

Normal

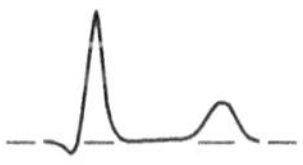

Figure 28.1 Normal T wave.

Peaked T wave

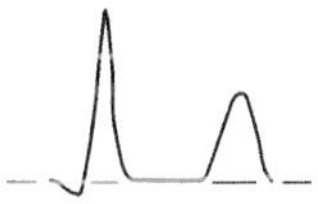

Figure 28.2 Peaked T wave.

Degrees of ST segment elevation

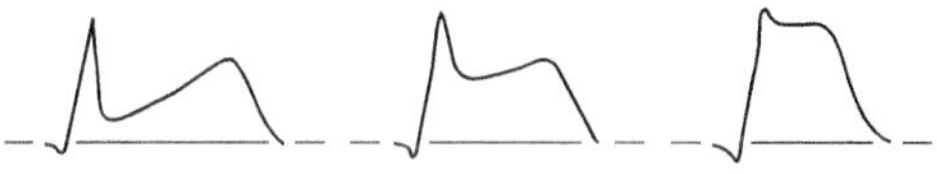

Figure 28.3 Degree of ST segment elevation.

Medical Student Survival Skills: ECG, First Edition. Philip Jevon and Jayant Gupta.
© 2020 John Wiley & Sons Ltd. Published 2020 by John Wiley & Sons Ltd.
Companion website: www.wiley.com/go/jevon/medicalstudent

Hours to days following myocardial infarction

- In the leads facing the affected area there is loss of R waves and wide (>0.04 seconds or 1 small square) and deep (>0.2 mV or 2 small squares) Q waves may develop (Figure 28.4)
- ST elevation begins to subside and T waves become increasingly negative (Figure 28.5). The presence of deep and broad Q waves indicates there is necrosed myocardial tissue in the heart, which the leads face. The Q waves actually represent electrical activity in the opposite ventricular wall, which the leads view through an electrical window created by the necrosed (electrically inactive) myocardial tissue

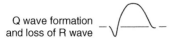

Q wave formation and loss of R wave

T wave inversion

Figure 28.4 Q wave formation and loss of R wave.   Figure 28.5 T wave inversion.

Days to weeks following myocardial infarction

- ST segment returns to the baseline and the T waves become more inverted and symmetrical. Sometimes the R wave completely disappears
- Most Q waves persist following a myocardial infarction

Localising the myocardial infarction from the ECG

- Inferior myocardial infarction: leads II, III, aVF
- Lateral myocardial infarction: leads I, aVL, V5, V6
- Anteroseptal myocardial infarction: V1, V2, V3
- Anterolateral myocardial infarction: V1, V2, V3, V4
- Posterior myocardial infarction: ECG changes can be seen indirectly in leads V1–V3 which face the endocardial surface of the posterior wall of the left ventricle; the 'mirror image' includes tall R waves, ST depression, and upright T waves

Reciprocal changes

- ST depression in leads remote from the site of the infarct are referred to as reciprocal changes. They are a highly sensitive indicator of acute myocardial infarction. They may be seen in leads that do not directly view the affected area of myocardium (they reflect a mirror image of their opposite leads). In Figure 28.3 ST elevation is evident in the inferior leads with reciprocal changes in the anterior leads. The depressed ST segments are typically horizontal or down-sloping

- Reciprocal changes are seen in approximately 70% of inferior and 30% of anterior myocardial infarctions
- Reciprocal changes in the anterior chest leads V1–V3 are sometimes evident in a posterior myocardial infarction

Diagnosing myocardial infarction in the presence of left bundle branch block

- Diagnosing myocardial infarction in the presence of left bundle branch block can be very difficult. Q waves, ST segment, and T wave changes can be obscured

ECG examples of myocardial infarction

- The ECG in Figure 28.6 displays the characteristic ECG changes associated with acute inferior myocardial infarction. ST elevation can clearly be seen in leads II, III, and aVF. Reciprocal changes can be seen, most markedly in the anterior leads (I, aVL, V2)

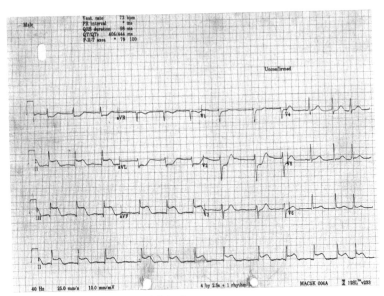

Figure 28.6 Acute inferior myocardial infarction.

- The ECG in Figure 28.7 displays the characteristic ECG changes associated with inferior myocardial infarction. There is ST elevation in the inferior leads (II, III, aVF). However, the T waves in these leads are beginning to become negative. This, with the development of Q waves in the inferior leads, is suggestive that the infarct is not acute. This patient was admitted with a 24 hour history of central chest pain
- The ECG in Figure 28.8 displays the characteristic ECG changes associated with posterior myocardial infarction. Tall R waves and reciprocal changes in anterior leads V1 and V2 and reciprocal changes in anterior leads I and aVL suggest this diagnosis. Posterior wall chest leads would be required to help confirm diagnosis of posterior myocardial infarction

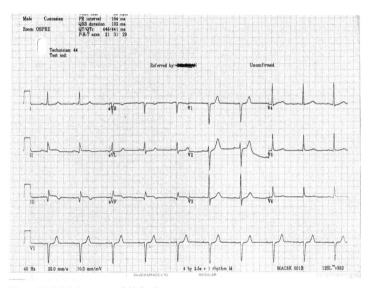

Figure 28.7 Inferior myocardial infarction.

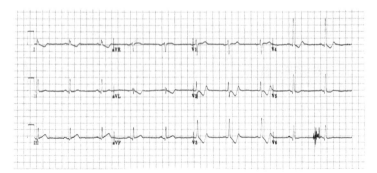

Figure 28.8 Posterior myocardial infarction: development of Q waves.

- The ECG in Figure 28.9 displays the characteristic ECG changes associated with anteroseptal or septal myocardial infarction. There is ST elevation in leads aVL and V1–V4. In addition there is right bundle branch block and left anterior fascicular block (bifascicular block), a complication of septal infarction. Regarding the right bundle branch block, the familiar rSR morphology has been replaced with QR morphology due to the infarction
- The ECG in Figure 28.10 displays the characteristic ECG changes associated with anterior myocardial infarction. The ST changes in the anterior leads (I, aVL, V2–V6) are hyperacute. This patient was admitted with a 1 hour history of chest pain

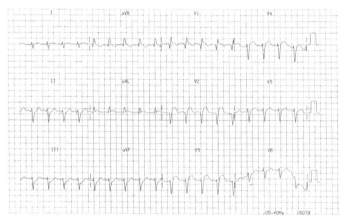

Figure 28.9 Acute posterior myocardial infarction.

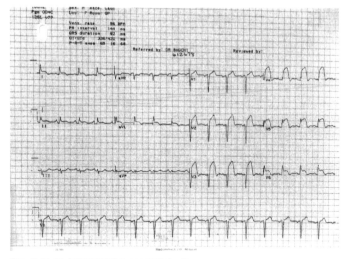

Figure 28.10 Anteroseptal myocardial infarction.

29 ECG changes associated with myocardial ischaemia

- Myocardial ischaemia can cause changes in the ST segment and T wave but not the QRS complex (except if it causes bundle branch block)
- Ischaemic changes associated with chest pain, but in the absence of myocardial infarction, are prognostically significant: 20% of patients with ST segment depression and 15% of patients with inverted T waves will experience severe angina, myocardial infarction, or death within 12 months of their initial presentation compared with 10% of patients with a normal trace

NB ST segment and T wave changes are not necessarily an indication of ischaemia; they can also be associated with left ventricular hypertrophy, digoxin toxicity, and hypokalaemia.

ST segment depression

- Myocardial ischaemia typically causes ST segment depression (Figure 29.1). In any given lead, the degree of ST segment depression is proportional to the size of the R wave, i.e. it is more prominent in leads V4–V6
- ECG changes associated with myocardial ischaemia (Figure 29.2): ST depression in the inferior (II, III, and aVL), and lateral (V4–V6) leads. This patient was complaining of severe chest pain when the 12 lead ECG was recorded

Medical Student Survival Skills: ECG, First Edition. Philip Jevon and Jayant Gupta.
© 2020 John Wiley & Sons Ltd. Published 2020 by John Wiley & Sons Ltd.
Companion website: www.wiley.com/go/jevon/medicalstudent

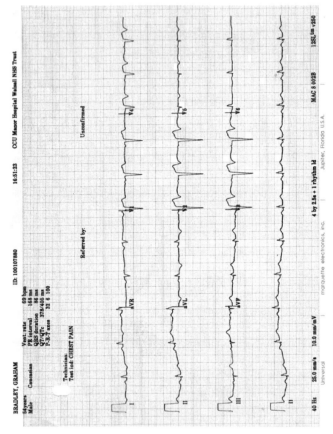

Figure 29.1 Anterolateral ischaemia.

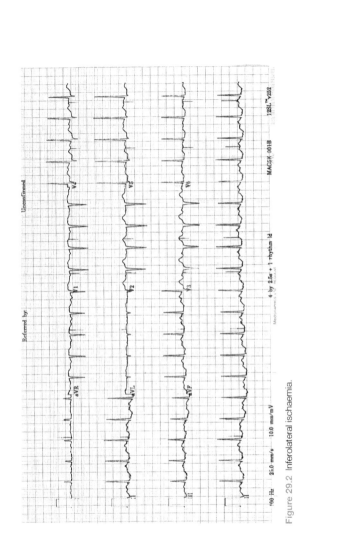

Figure 29.2 Inferolateral ischaemia.

T wave changes

T wave changes associated with myocardial ischaemia can present in a variety of different ways:

- Tall T waves: in leads V1–V3 may be due to posterior wall myocardial ischaemia (mirror image of T wave inversion)
- Biphasic T waves: particular seen in the anterior chest leads
- Inverted T waves (NB T waves are normally inverted in leads III, aVR, and V1)
- Flattened T waves

ECG changes associated with bundle branch block

Left bundle branch block (figure 30.1)

- Conduction down the left bundle branches is blocked
- Most commonly caused by ischaemic heart disease, hypertensive disease, or dilated cardiomyopathy
- Rare for left bundle branch block to be present in the absence of organic disease
- Diagnosis can be made by examining chest leads V1 and V6

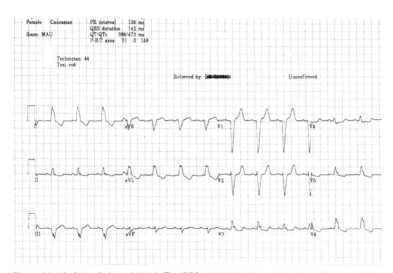

Figure 30.1 Left bundle branch block. The QRS width is 0.16 seconds or 4 small squares. The W-shaped morphology of the QRS complex in V1 and the M-shaped morphology of the QRS complex in V6 can be seen clearly.

Medical Student Survival Skills: ECG, First Edition. Philip Jevon and Jayant Gupta.
© 2020 John Wiley & Sons Ltd. Published 2020 by John Wiley & Sons Ltd.
Companion website: www.wiley.com/go/jevon/medicalstudent

ECG changes associated with left bundle branch block

- Septal depolarisation occurs from right to left: small Q wave in V1 and R wave in V6 (the direction of intraventricular depolarisation is reversed, the septal waves are lost and are replaced with R waves)
- Right ventricular depolarisation first: R wave in V1 and S wave in V6 (often appearing as just a notch)
- Left ventricular depolarisation second: S wave in V1 and R wave in V6
- Delay in ventricular depolarisation leads to a wide (0.12 seconds or 3 small squares or more) QRS complex
- Abnormal depolarisation of the ventricles leads to secondary repolarisation changes: ST segment depression together with T wave inversion in leads with a dominant R wave; ST segment elevation and upright T waves in leads with a dominant S wave (i.e. discordance between the QRS complex and ST segment and T wave)
- Left bundle branch block is best viewed in V6: the QRS complex is wide and has an M-shaped configuration. The W-shaped QRS appearance in V1 is seldom seen

Right bundle branch block (figure 30.2)

- Conduction down the right bundle branch is blocked
- Conditions associated with right bundle branch block include ischaemic heart disease, pulmonary embolism, rheumatic heart disease, and cardiomyopathy
- Diagnosis can be made by examining chest leads V1 and V6

ECG changes associated with right bundle branch block

- Septal depolarisation occurs from left to right as normal: small R wave in V1 and small Q wave in V6
- Left ventricular depolarisation first: S wave in V1 and R wave in V6
- Right ventricular depolarisation second: a second R wave in V1 and a deep wide S wave in V6
- Latter part of the QRS complex is abnormal: slurred R and S waves in V1 and V6, respectively
- ST segment depression and T wave inversion in the right precordial leads
- Right bundle branch block is best viewed in V1: the QRS complex is wide (0.12 s/3 small squares or more) and has a characteristic rSR pattern

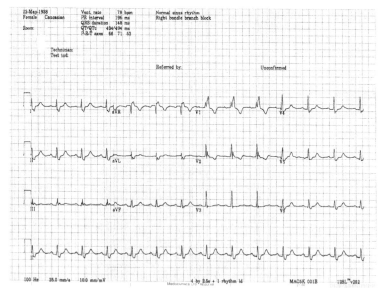

Figure 30.2 Right bundle branch block. The QRS width is 0.12 seconds or 3 small squares. The rSR W-shaped morphology of the QRS complex in V1 and the M-shaped morphology of the QRS complex in V6 can be seen clearly.

Left anterior fascicular block

- Sometimes termed left anterior hemiblock
- Conduction down the anterior fascicle of the left bundle branch is blocked
- Depolarisation of the left ventricle is via the left posterior fascicle. The cardiac axis therefore rotates in an upwards direction resulting in left axis deviation
- Left anterior fascicular block is characterised by a mean frontal plane axis more leftward than 30° in the absence of inferior myocardial infarction or other cause of left axis deviation

Left posterior fascicular block

- Sometimes termed left posterior hemiblock
- Conduction down the posterior fascicle of the left bundle branch is blocked
- Depolarisation of the left ventricle is via the left anterior fascicle. The cardiac axis therefore rotates in a downwards direction resulting in right axis deviation
- Left posterior fascicular block is characterised by a mean frontal plane axis of greater than 90° in the absence of another cause of right axis deviation

Bifascicular block (figure 30.3)

- Right bundle branch block and blockage of either the left anterior or posterior fascicle (determined by the presence of left or right axis deviation, respectively). Right bundle branch block together with left anterior fascicular block is the commonest type of bifascicular block
- Bifascicular block is indicative of widespread conduction problems
  The ECG in Figure 30.3 displays bifascicular block; there is right bundle branch block and left anterior fascicular block (left axis deviation).

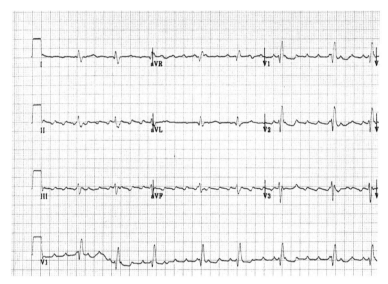

Figure 30.3 Bifascicular block.

Trifascicular block (figure 30.4)

- Bifascicular block and first degree AV block
- Third degree AV block will ensue if the other fascicle fails as well

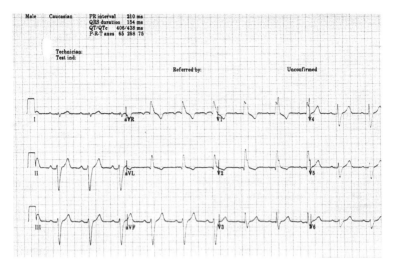

Figure 30.4 Trifascicular block.

31 Wolff–Parkinson–White syndrome

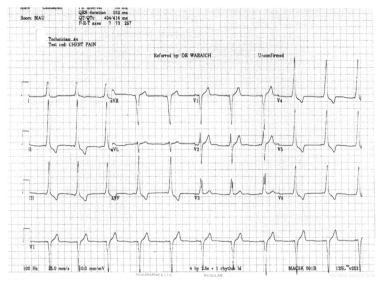

Figure 31.1 Wolff–Parkinson–White syndrome.

- Wolff–Parkinson–White (WPW) syndrome is a condition where atrial impulses bypass the AV junction and activate the ventricular myocardium directly via an accessory pathway (bundle of Kent)
- More than one accessory pathway is present in 10% of cases
- The accessory pathway(s) allows the formation of a re-entry circuit, which can give rise to either a narrow complex or a broad complex tachycardia depending on whether the AV junction or the accessory pathway is used for antegrade conduction
- WPW syndrome is the commonest cause of an AV re-entrant tachycardia. Thought to be hereditary, its incidence is 0.1–0.3% of the population

Medical Student Survival Skills: ECG, First Edition. Philip Jevon and Jayant Gupta.
© 2020 John Wiley & Sons Ltd. Published 2020 by John Wiley & Sons Ltd.
Companion website: www.wiley.com/go/jevon/medicalstudent

Identifying ECG features

- Short PR interval (<0.12 seconds or 3 small squares)
- Wide QRS complex (>0.12 seconds or 3 small squares) with an initial delta wave and paroxysmal tachycardia
- In sinus rhythm the atrial impulse is conducted rapidly down to the ventricles via the accessory pathway (it is not subjected to the normal delay as would be encountered in the AV node) – hence the short PR interval. However, once the impulse reaches the ventricular myocardium, initially it is conducted (slowly) through non-specialised conduction tissue, distorting the early part of the R wave producing the characteristic delta wave

Classification

The WPW syndrome is traditionally classified into two types (A and B) according to the ECG morphology of in leads V1 and V2.
- *Type A*: left-sided pathway resulting in a predominant R wave
- *Type B*: right-sided pathway resulting in a predominant S or QS wave

Complications

- The frequency of paroxysmal tachycardia associated with WPW syndrome increases with age
- If atrial fibrillation is present the ventricular response depends on the antegrade refractory period of the accessory pathway and may exceed $300\,min^{-1}$, resulting in ventricular fibrillation and cardiac arrest

Treatment

- Patients who are symptomatic (palpitations or syncope) should be referred for electrophysiology studies
- Catheter ablation has a high success rate
- Drugs that block the AV junction, e.g. digoxin, verapamil, and adenosine, are particularly dangerous in WPW syndrome in the presence of atrial fibrillation and should be avoided (they decrease the refractoriness of the accessory pathways and increase the frequency of conduction, resulting in a rapid ventricular response that may lead to ventricular fibrillation)

Appendix A: Resuscitation council (UK) bradycardia algorithm

Medical Student Survival Skills: ECG, First Edition. Philip Jevon and Jayant Gupta.
© 2020 John Wiley & Sons Ltd. Published 2020 by John Wiley & Sons Ltd.
Companion website: www.wiley.com/go/jevon/medicalstudent

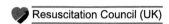

Resuscitation Council (UK)

2010 Resuscitation Guidelines

Adult bradycardia algorithm

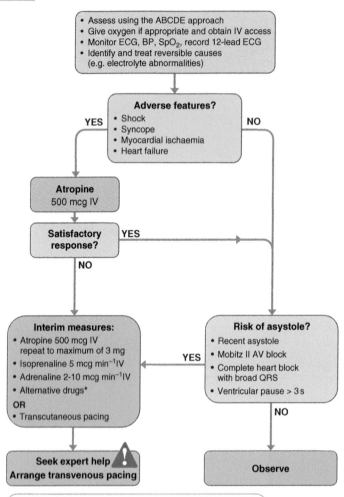

- Assess using the ABCDE approach
- Give oxygen if appropriate and obtain IV access
- Monitor ECG, BP, SpO$_2$, record 12-lead ECG
- Identify and treat reversible causes
  (e.g. electrolyte abnormalities)

Adverse features?

YES   • Shock   NO
- Syncope
- Myocardial ischaemia
- Heart failure

Atropine
500 mcg IV

Satisfactory response?   YES

NO

Interim measures:
- Atropine 500 mcg IV
  repeat to maximum of 3 mg
- Isoprenaline 5 mcg min^{-1}IV
- Adrenaline 2-10 mcg min^{-1}IV
- Alternative drugs*

OR
- Transcutaneous pacing

YES

Risk of asystole?
- Recent asystole
- Mobitz II AV block
- Complete heart block
  with broad QRS
- Ventricular pause > 3 s

NO

Seek expert help
Arrange transvenous pacing

Observe

*Alternatives include:
- Aminophylline
- Dopamine
- Glucagon (if beta-blocker or calcium channel blocker overdose)
- Glycopyrrolate can be used instead of atropine

Appendix B: Resuscitation council (UK) tachycardia algorithm

Medical Student Survival Skills: ECG, First Edition. Philip Jevon and Jayant Gupta.
© 2020 John Wiley & Sons Ltd. Published 2020 by John Wiley & Sons Ltd.
Companion website: www.wiley.com/go/jevon/medicalstudent

Resuscitation Council (UK)

Resuscitation Guidelines

2010

Adult tachycardia (with pulse) algorithm

- Assess using the ABCDE approach
- Give oxygen if appropriate and obtain IV access
- Monitor ECG, BP, SpO₂, record 12-lead ECG
- Identify and treat reversible causes (e.g. electrolyte abnormalities)

Adverse features?
- Shock
- Syncope
- Myocardial ischaemia
- Heart failure

Yes / Unstable

Synchronised DC Shock
Up to 3 attempts

- Amiodarone 300 mg IV over 10-20 min and repeat shock; followed by:
- Amiodarone 900 mg over 24 h

No / Stable

Is QRS narrow (< 0.12 s)?

Broad

Broad QRS
Is rhythm regular?

Irregular

Seek expert help

Possibilities include:
- **AF with bundle branch block** treat as for narrow complex
- **Pre-excited AF** consider amiodarone
- **Polymorphic VT** (e.g. torsade de pointes - give magnesium 2 g over 10 min)

Regular

If **ventricular tachycardia** (or uncertain rhythm):
- Amiodarone 300 mg IV over 20-60 min; then 900 mg over 24 h

If previously confirmed **SVT with bundle branch block:**
- Give adenosine as for regular narrow complex tachycardia

Narrow

Narrow QRS
Is rhythm regular?

Regular

- Use vagal manoeuvres
- Adenosine 6 mg rapid IV bolus; if unsuccessful give 12 mg; if unsuccessful give further 12 mg.
- Monitor ECG continuously

Sinus rhythm restored?

Yes

Probable **re-entry paroxysmal SVT:**
- Record 12-lead ECG in sinus rhythm
- If recurs, give adenosine again & consider choice of anti-arrhythmic prophylaxis

No

Seek expert help

Possible **atrial flutter**
- Control rate (e.g. β-Blocker)

Irregular

Irregular Narrow Complex Tachycardia
Probable atrial fibrillation
Control rate with:
- β-Blocker or diltiazem
- Consider digoxin or amiodarone if evidence of heart failure

Appendix C: Resuscitation council (UK) advanced life support (ALS) algorithm

Medical Student Survival Skills: ECG, First Edition. Philip Jevon and Jayant Gupta.
© 2020 John Wiley & Sons Ltd. Published 2020 by John Wiley & Sons Ltd.
Companion website: www.wiley.com/go/jevon/medicalstudent

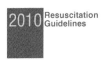

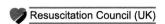

Adult Advanced Life Support

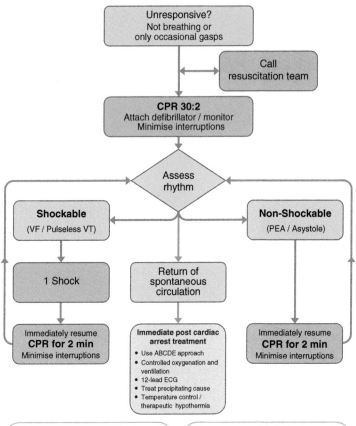

Appendix D: Vagal manoeuvres

- If there are no contraindications, vagal manoeuvres can be used to help terminate a tachyarrhythmia, e.g. narrow complex tachycardia
- They are used to stimulate the vagus nerve and induce a reflex slowing of the heart
- Successful in terminating 25% of narrow complex tachycardias
- Caution should be exercised regarding the use of vagal manoeuvres. Profound vagal tone can induce sudden bradycardia and trigger ventricular fibrillation, particularly in the presence of digitalis toxicity or acute cardiac ischaemia
- Carotid sinus massage should not be used in the presence of a carotid bruit as atheromatous plaque rupture could embolise into the cerebral circulation causing a cerebrovascular accident; elderly patients are more vulnerable to plaque rupture and cerebrovascular complications

 NB When performing carotid sinus massage: only massage the one side (massaging both sides together could cause asystole).

- Valsalva manoeuvre: forced expiration against a closed glottis, e.g. ask the patient to blow into a 20 ml syringe with enough force to push the plunger back

Medical Student Survival Skills: ECG, First Edition. Philip Jevon and Jayant Gupta.
© 2020 John Wiley & Sons Ltd. Published 2020 by John Wiley & Sons Ltd.
Companion website: www.wiley.com/go/jevon/medicalstudent

Appendix E: Synchronised electrical cardioversion

- Synchronised electrical cardioversion is a reliable method of converting a tachyarrhythmia to sinus rhythm
- Due to the associated risks, e.g. ventricular fibrillation or stroke, it is generally only undertaken when pharmacological cardioversion has been unsuccessful or if adverse signs are present, e.g. chest pain, hypotension, reduced level of consciousness, rapid ventricular rate, and dyspnoea

Synchronisation with the R wave

- The shock must be delivered on the R wave, not the T wave, as delivery of the shock during the refractory period of the cardiac cycle (T wave) could induce ventricular fibrillation
- The defibrillator must therefore be synchronised with the patient's ECG

 Common misinterpretations and pitfalls

Synchronisation with the R wave: it is easy to forget that it is usually necessary to re-synchronise the defibrillator after a synchronised shock is delivered.

Shock energies

- Follow local protocols
- Broad complex tachycardia and atrial fibrillation: 120–150 J biphasic (200 J monophasic) is recommended initially
- Regular narrow complex tachycardia or atrial flutter: 70–120 J biphasic (100 J monophasic) is recommended initially

Medical Student Survival Skills: ECG, First Edition. Philip Jevon and Jayant Gupta.
© 2020 John Wiley & Sons Ltd. Published 2020 by John Wiley & Sons Ltd.
Companion website: www.wiley.com/go/jevon/medicalstudent

Procedure

- Record a 12 lead ECG, unless the patient is severely compromised and doing so will delay the procedure
- Explain the procedure to the patient. Consent should be obtained if possible. If the patient is not unconscious, they must be anaesthetised or sedated for the procedure
- Ensure the resuscitation equipment is immediately available
- Establish ECG monitoring using the defibrillator that will be used for cardioversion
- Select an ECG monitoring lead that will provide a clear ECG trace, e.g. lead II
- Press the 'synch' button on the defibrillator
- Check the ECG trace to ensure that only the R waves are being synchronised, i.e. a 'synchronised' dot or arrow should appear on each R wave and nowhere else on the PQRST cycle, e.g. on tall T waves
- Prepare the chest: dry it and shave if necessary
- Apply large adhesive electrodes to the patient's chest, one just to the right of the sternum, below the right clavicle, and the other in the mid-axillary line, approximately level with the V6 ECG electrode or female breast
- Select the appropriate energy level on the defibrillator (see earlier for recommended levels)
- Charge the defibrillator and shout 'stand clear'
- Check all personnel are safely clear prior to defibrillation. No person should be touching the patient or anything in contact with the patient, e.g. bed, drip stand
- Ensure oxygen is remove at least 1 m away from the patient
- Check the ECG monitor to ensure that the patient is still in the tachyarrhythmia that requires cardioversion, that the synchronised button remains activated and that it is still synchronising with the R waves
- Press shock button to discharge the shock. There is usually a slight delay between pressing the shock button and shock discharge
- Re-assess the ECG trace. The 'synch' button will usually need to be reactivated if further cardioversion is required (on some defibrillators it is necessary to actually switch off the 'synch' button if further cardioversion is not indicated). Stepwise increases in energy will be required if cardioversion needs to be repeated
- After successful cardioversion, record a 12 lead ECG
- Monitor the patient's vital signs until they have fully recovered from the anaesthetic or sedative

OSCE Key Learning Points

Key safety precautions: Electrical cardioversion

✔ ECG monitoring: synchronisation on R wave

✔ Patient sedated

✔ Resuscitation equipment and advanced life support (ALS) trained personnel present

✔ Atrial fibrillation: need for anticoagulation?

Appendix F: External (transcutaneous) pacing

Indications

- Profound bradycardia, e.g. sometimes found in complete heart block, that has not responded to pharmacological treatment, e.g. atropine

 NB If the intrinsic QRS complexes are not associated with a pulse (pulseless electrical activity or PEA), attempts at pacing will be futile.

- Ventricular standstill: P waves (atrial contraction) only on the ECG

Advantages

- Can be quickly established
- Easy to undertake, minimal training
- Risks associated with central venous cannulation are avoided
- Can be undertaken by nurses

Medical Student Survival Skills: ECG, First Edition. Philip Jevon and Jayant Gupta.
© 2020 John Wiley & Sons Ltd. Published 2020 by John Wiley & Sons Ltd.
Companion website: www.wiley.com/go/jevon/medicalstudent

Appendix G: Procedure for transcutaneous pacing

- If appropriate, explain the procedure to the patient
- Ideally, first remove excess chest hair from the pacing electrode sites by clipping close to the patient's skin using a pair of scissors (shaving the skin is not recommended as any nicks in the skin can lead to burns and pain during pacing)
- Attach the pacing electrodes following the manufacturer's instructions
- Pacing-only electrodes: attach the anterior electrode on the left anterior chest, midway between the xiphoid process and the left nipple (V2–V3 ECG electrode position) and attach the posterior electrode below the left scapula, lateral to the spine and at the same level as the anterior electrode – this anterior/posterior configuration will ensure that the position of the electrodes does not interfere with defibrillation
- Multifunctional electrodes (pacing and defibrillation): place the anterior electrode below the right clavicle and the lateral electrode in the mid-axillary line lateral to the left nipple (V6 ECG electrode position) – this anterolateral position is convenient during cardiopulmonary resuscitation (CPR) as chest compressions do not have to be interrupted
- Check that the pacing electrodes and connecting cables are applied following the manufacturer's recommendations: if they are reversed, pacing may either be ineffective or high capture thresholds may be required
- Adjust the ECG gain (size) accordingly. This will help ensure that the intrinsic QRS complexes are sensed
- Select demand mode on the pacing unit on the defibrillator
- Select an appropriate rate for external pacing, usually 60–90 min^{-1}
- Set the pacing current at the lowest level, turn on the pacemaker unit and while observing both the patient and the ECG, gradually increase the current until electrical capture occurs (QRS complexes following the pacing spike). Electrical capture usually occurs when the current delivered is in the range of 50–100 mA

Medical Student Survival Skills: ECG, First Edition. Philip Jevon and Jayant Gupta.
© 2020 John Wiley & Sons Ltd. Published 2020 by John Wiley & Sons Ltd.
Companion website: www.wiley.com/go/jevon/medicalstudent

- Check the patient's pulse. If they have a palpable pulse (mechanical capture), request expert help and prepare for transvenous pacing. If there is no pulse, start CPR. If there is good electrical capture, but no mechanical capture, this is indicative of a non-viable myocardium. Note that there is no electrical hazard if in contact with the patient during pacing

Appendix H: Definitions

Aberrant conduction: conduction of the supraventricular impulse to the ventricles with a bundle branch block pattern

Automaticity: inherent ability of automatic or pacemaker cells to initiate electrical impulses

Bradycardia: heart rate <60 bpm

Cardiac arrhythmia: literally, total lack of rhythm; although used to describe any cardiac rhythm that deviates from sinus rhythm

Depolarisation: electrical discharging of the cell (P waves and QRS complexes)

Ectopic: literally an abnormal place or position (Greek word 'ektopos' meaning 'out of place'). The terms ectopic beat, premature beat (atrial premature beats or APBs), and extrasystole are synonymous

Electrocardiogram (ECG): a record or display, produced by electrocardiography, of the electrical activity in the heart

Electrocardiograph: a device that records the electrical activity in the heart, e.g. cardiac monitor or ECG machine

Morphology: shape of QRS complex

Repolarisation: electrical recharging of the cell (T waves)

Tachycardia: heart rate >100 bpm

Medical Student Survival Skills: ECG, First Edition. Philip Jevon and Jayant Gupta.
© 2020 John Wiley & Sons Ltd. Published 2020 by John Wiley & Sons Ltd.
Companion website: www.wiley.com/go/jevon/medicalstudent

References

Fuster, V., Rydén, L.E., Cannom, D.S. et al. (2006). ACC/AHA/ESC 2006 guidelines for the management of patients with atrial fibrillation: A report of the American College of Cardiology/American Heart Association Task Force on Practice Guidelines and the European Society of Cardiology Committee for Practice Guidelines (Writing Committee to Revise the 2001 Guidelines for the Management of Patients With Atrial Fibrillation): Developed in collaboration with the European Heart Rhythm Association and the Heart Rhythm Society. *Circulation* 114: e257–e354.

Resuscitation Council (UK) (2018). *Adult Advanced Life Support*. London: Resuscitation Council (UK) www.resus.org.uk (accessed November 2018.

McWilliam, J. (1889). Electrical stimulation of the heart in man. *BMJ;* 1: 348.

Index

Note: Page numbers in *italics* refer to figures.
Page numbers in **bold** refer to tables.

Medical Student Survival Skills: ECG, First Edition. Philip Jevon and Jayant Gupta.
© 2020 John Wiley & Sons Ltd. Published 2020 by John Wiley & Sons Ltd.
Companion website: www.wiley.com/go/jevon/medicalstudent